Tendon Repair and Reconstruction

Editors

JIN BO TANG
STEVE K. LEE

HAND CLINICS

www.hand.theclinics.com

Consulting Editor
KEVIN C. CHUNG

May 2013 • Volume 29 • Number 2

ELSEVIER

1600 John F. Kennedy Boulevard • Suite 1800 • Philadelphia, Pennsylvania, 19103-2899

http://www.theclinics.com

HAND CLINICS Volume 29, Number 2
May 2013 ISSN 0749-0712, ISBN-13: 978-1-4557-7097-7

Editor: Jennifer Flynn-Briggs

Hand Clinics (ISSN 0749-0712) is published quarterly by Elsevier Inc., 360 Park Avenue South, New York, NY 10010-1710. Months of publication are February, May, August, and November. Business and Editorial Offices: 1600 John F. Kennedy Blvd., Ste. 1800, Philadelphia, PA 19103-2899. Customer Service Office: 3251 Riverport Lane, Maryland Heights, MO 63043. Periodicals postage paid at New York, NY and at additional mailing offices. Subscription price is $368.00 per year (domestic individuals), $583.00 per year (domestic institutions), $184.00 per year (domestic students/residents), $420.00 per year (Canadian individuals), $666.00 per year (Canadian institutions), $500.00 per year (international individuals), $666.00 per year (international institutions), and $243.00 per year (international and Canadian students/residents). Foreign air speed delivery is included in all *Clinics* subscription prices. All prices are subject to change without notice. **POSTMASTER:** Send address changes to *Hand Clinics*, Elsevier Health Sciences Division, Subscription Customer Service, 3251 Riverport Lane, Maryland Heights, MO 63043. Customer Service (orders, claims, online, change of address): Elsevier Health Sciences Division, Subscription Customer Service, 3251 Riverport Lane, Maryland Heights, MO 63043. Tel: 1-800-654-2452 (U.S. and Canada); 314-447-8871 (outside U.S. and Canada). Fax: 314-447-8029. E-mail: journalscustomerservice-usa@elsevier.com (for print support); journalsonlinesupport-usa@elsevier.com (for online support).

Reprints. For copies of 100 or more of articles in this publication, please contact the Commercial Reprints Department, Elsevier Inc., 360 Park Avenue South, New York, New York 10010-1710. Tel.: 212-633-3812; Fax: 212-462-1935; E-mail: reprints@elsevier.com.

Hand Clinics is covered in *MEDLINE/PubMed (Index Medicus), Current Contents/Clinical Medicine, EMBASE/Excerpta Medica,* and *ISI/BIOMED.*

Printed and bound by CPI Group (UK) Ltd, Croydon, CR0 4YY

Transferred to Digital Printing, 2013

Contributors

CONSULTING EDITOR

KEVIN C. CHUNG, MD
Charles B.G. de Nancrede Professor of Surgery, Section of Plastic Surgery, Department of Surgery, Assistant Dean for Faculty Affairs, Associate Director of Global REACH, University of Michigan Medical School, The University of Michigan Health System, Ann Arbor, Michigan

EDITORS

JIN BO TANG, MD
Professor and Chair, Department of Hand Surgery, Chair, The Hand Surgery Research Center, Affiliated Hospital of Nantong University, Nantong, Jiangsu, China

STEVE K. LEE, MD
Associate Professor, Hand and Upper Extremity Service, Department of Orthopaedic Surgery, Hospital for Special Surgery, New York, New York

AUTHORS

PETER C. AMADIO, MD
Lloyd A and Barbara A Amundson Professor of Orthopedic Surgery, Mayo Clinic, Rochester, Minnesota

PHILIP E. BLAZAR, MD
Associate Professor, Department of Orthopedic Surgery, Brigham and Women's Hospital, Harvard Medical School, Boston, Massachusetts

MARTIN I. BOYER, MD
Carol B. and Jerome T. Loeb Professor of Orthopedic Surgery, Department of Orthopedic Surgery, Washington University, St Louis, Missouri

MATTHEW J. CARTY, MD
Assistant Professor, Division of Plastic Surgery, Brigham and Women's Hospital, Harvard Medical School, Boston, Massachusetts

SEAN P. CLANCY, OTR/L, CHT
Program coordinator, Hand Therapy, Senior Faculty, Physical Therapy Orthopedic Residency Program, University of Chicago Medicine, Therapy Services, Chicago, Illinois

AARON DALUISKI, MD
Division of Hand and Upper Extremity Surgery, Department of Orthopaedic Surgery, Hospital for Special Surgery, New York, New York

SÉBASTIEN DURAND, MD, PhD
Hand Surgery and Peripheral Nerve Surgery, Groupe Main Provence, Aix-en-Provence, France

CHRISTOPHER J. DY, MD, MSPH
Division of Hand and Upper Extremity Surgery, Department of Orthopaedic Surgery, Hospital for Special Surgery, New York, New York

DAVID ELLIOT, MA, FRCS
Consultant Hand Surgeon, Hand Surgery Department, St Andrew's Centre for Plastic Surgery, Broomfield Hospital, Chelmsford, Essex, United Kingdom

THOMAS GIESEN, MD
Consultant Hand Surgeon, Hand Surgery Department, St Andrew's Centre for Plastic Surgery, Broomfield Hospital, Chelmsford, Essex, United Kingdom

STEVEN M. GREEN, MD
Associate Clinical Professor of Orthopaedic Surgery, New York University and Mount Sinai Schools of Medicine; Associate Chief, Division of Hand Surgery, Hospital for Joint Diseases, New York University, New York, New York

DONALD H. LALONDE, MD, FRCSC
Department of Surgery, Saint John Regional Hospital, Professor of Surgery, Dalhousie University, Saint John, Canada

STEVE K. LEE, MD
Associate Professor, Hand and Upper Extremity Service, Department of Orthopaedic Surgery, Hospital for Special Surgery, New York, New York

ALISON L. MARTIN, BSc
Department of Surgery, Saint John Regional Hospital, Dalhousie University, Saint John, Canada; Faculty of Medicine, Dalhousie University, Halifax, Nova Scotia, Canada

DANIEL P. MASS, MD
Professor of Surgery, Department of Orthopaedic Surgery and Rehabilitation Medicine, Vice-Chairman, Orthopaedic Surgery, Pritzker School of Medicine, University of Chicago; Director, Hand and Microsurgery Fellowship Program, University of Chicago Medicine, Chicago, Illinois

KIERAN O'SHEA, MB, FRCSI
Consultant Orthopaedic Surgeon, St Vincents University Hospital, Elm Park, Dublin, Ireland

MARTIN A. POSNER, MD
Clinical Professor of Orthopaedic Surgery, New York University School of Medicine; Chief, Division of Hand Surgery, Hospital for Joint Diseases, New York University, New York, New York

LAUREN ROSENBLATT, BS
Hand and Upper Extremity Service, Department of Orthopaedic Surgery, Hospital for Special Surgery, New York, New York

MICHAEL SANDOW, FRCS
Director, Hand and Upper Limb Service, Department of Orthopedics and Trauma; Physiotherapy Department, Royal Adelaide Hospital, Adelaide, Australia

ROBERT SAVAGE, MS, FRCS
Consultant, Trauma and Orthopedic Department, Royal Gwent Hospital, Newport, Gwent, United Kingdom

LAURA-CARMEN SITA-ALB, MD
Plastic Surgery and Reconstructive Microsurgery, Groupe Main Provence, Aix-en-Provence, France

JIN BO TANG, MD
Professor and Chair, Department of Hand Surgery, Chair, The Hand Surgery Research Center, Affiliated Hospital of Nantong University, Nantong, Jiangsu, China

SCOTT W. WOLFE, MD
Attending Orthopaedic Surgeon, Chief Emeritus of the Hand and Upper Extremity Service, Hospital for Special Surgery, Director, Center for Brachial Plexus and Traumatic Nerve Injury; Professor of Orthopedic Surgery, Weill Cornell Medical College, New York, New York

YA FANG WU, MD
Lecturer, Department of Hand Surgery, The Hand Surgery Research Center, Affiliated Hospital of Nantong University, Nantong, Jiangsu, China

CHUNFENG ZHAO, MD
Associate Professor, Department of Orthopedics, Mayo Clinic, Rochester, Minnesota

Contents

Gliding Resistance and Modifications of Gliding Surface of Tendon: Clinical Perspectives   **159**

Peter C. Amadio

> The smooth gliding of the normal human digital flexor is maintained by synovial fluid lubrication and lubricants bound to the tendon surface. This system can be disrupted by degenerative conditions such as trigger finger, or by trauma. The resistance to tendon gliding after surgical repair of the lacerated digital flexor tendon relates to location of suture knots, exposure of suture materials, and type of surgical repair and materials. Restoration of a functioning gliding surface after injury can be helped by using low-friction, high-strength suture designs, therapy that enables gliding, and the addition of lubricants to the tendon surface.

Tendon Healing, Edema, and Resistance to Flexor Tendon Gliding: Clinical Implications   **167**

Ya Fang Wu and Jin Bo Tang

> Early flexor tendon healing is characterized by peak cellular apoptosis of both inflammatory and tendon cells in the first week, followed by progressively greater tenocyte proliferation in the second and third weeks. Tenocyte apoptosis is a predominant event, but proliferation of tenocytes is minimal in the middle and late healing periods. Edematous subcutaneous tissues, edema of the tendon, the intact annular pulleys, and extensor tendons all greatly contribute to the resistance. Careful consideration of the contributing factors and dynamics offers insight into strategies to reduce repair rupture and maximize tendon gliding through surgery and postoperative motion protocols.

Current Practice of Primary Flexor Tendon Repair: A Global View   **179**

Jin Bo Tang, Peter C. Amadio, Martin I. Boyer, Robert Savage, Chunfeng Zhao, Michael Sandow, Steve K. Lee, and Scott W. Wolfe

> In this article, a group of international leaders in tendon surgery of the hand provide details of their current methods of primary flexor tendon repair. They are from recognized hand centers around the world, from which major contributions to the development of methods for flexor tendon repair have come over the past 2 decades. Changes made since the early 1990s regarding surgical methods and postoperative care for the flexor tendon repair are also discussed. Current practice methods used in the leading hand centers are summarized, and key points in providing the best possible clinical outcomes are outlined.

pain, or dysfunction after attempted nonoperative management of a single pulley rupture, or during concurrent or staged flexor tendon repair or reconstruction. If the pulley cannot be repaired primarily, pulley reconstruction can be performed using graft woven into remnant pulley rim or looping graft around the phalanx. Regardless of the reconstructive technique, the surgeon should emulate the length, tension, and glide of the native pulley.

Whether it is a primary or a delayed flexor digitorum profundus (FDP) repair, no general consent has been found, and no perfect treatment has been imposed. The authors utilize 2 new techniques for FDP reconstruction that allow immediate postoperative mobilization and excellent functional outcome. Harvesting of the donor hemi tendon, both FDP and flexor digitorum superficialis, is the closest match in terms of muscle agonism and excursion, and does not result in an imbalance of forces across the donor joint with the potential complications that this may create.

This article reviews recent reports of outcomes of flexor tendon repair and discusses the problems associated with such surgeries. Reports of no repair rupture in individual case series have emerged recently. Their results move toward the clinical goal of primary repair without repair rupture. The Strickland method remains the most common to record the outcomes. Outcomes should be provided by subzones of the tendon injuries, and the level of expertise of the surgeons expertise should be reported to allow comparisons of the results.

Extensor tendon injuries occur frequently. An in-depth understanding of the intricate anatomy of the extensor mechanism is necessary to guide management. Careful counseling is helpful in ensuring patient compliance and optimal outcomes for nonoperative and surgical treatments. For distal lacerations in Zones II-V, we prefer the running-interlocked horizontal mattress technique. Prolonged immobilization or inadvertent shortening of the extensor mechanism can create the unintended consequence of joint stiffness. While clinical outcomes have improved with modern repairs and rehabilitation, patients should be advised that a slight extensor lag may persist and full flexion may not be possible despite seemingly successful treatment.

Injuries to the finger extensor apparatus are very common and may produce chronic deformity and loss of function. Diagnosis is contingent on an understanding of the complex anatomy of this region as well as the ability to perform a careful physical examination. Immobilization is usually the most effective treatment of acute problems. Surgery is often necessary for chronic conditions, but the results are much less predictably corrective.

HAND CLINICS

Erratum

An error was made in the November 2012 issue of Hand Clinics (28:4) on page 493 in "Free Vascularized Medial Femoral Condyle Autograft for Challenging Upper Extremity Nonunions" by David B. Jones Jr, Peter C. Rhee, Allen T. Bishop, and Alexander Y. Shin. Dr Bishop's first name was spelled incorrectly. Allen is the correct spelling.

Hand Clin 29 (2013) xi
http://dx.doi.org/10.1016/j.hcl.2013.03.005

Preface

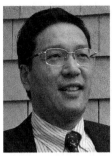 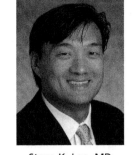

Jin Bo Tang, MD   Steve K. Lee, MD
Editors

It is a great pleasure and honor to edit this issue of *Hand Clinics* to which a worldwide group of distinguished experts on tendon repair and reconstruction has contributed. This issue starts with reviews from 2 research units whose work in the past decade has reshaped our understanding of tendon repair with regard to resistance to tendon motion. These basic science findings set the stage for current surgical practices and postoperative care. The next 3 articles present first a global view of current practice, followed by detailed description of methods and recommendations of 2 master hand surgeons: Dr. David Elliot on his experience and outcomes over 3 decades of primary flexor tendon repair and Dr. Don Lalonde on his innovative "wide-awake" primary flexor tendon repair. The late half of this issue is devoted to secondary flexor tendon repair and complex extensor tendon repair. These topics have perplexed hand surgeons for decades, and here, a panel of experts has summarized their preferred methods—from secondary pulley and tendon reconstruction to treatment in complex hand injury—to tackle these problems. The final article, a summary on postoperative care and rehabilitation, gives an overview on evolving methods and concepts of the care after surgery.

The inaugural issue of *Hand Clinics* in 1985 was devoted to the tendon repair. Flexor tendon repair was the theme of a 2005 issue of *Hand Clinics.* Tendon surgery has evolved rapidly in the past 30 years. The readers will find that the techniques and concepts have been evolved even from practices seen a decade ago. Our goal of treatment, however, remains the same: to achieve best possible treatment outcomes. Tendon surgery is a fundamental yet one of the most difficult areas of hand surgery. Desired outcomes heavily rely on precision of surgery and rehabilitation. With this consideration in mind, we tried to offer readers detailed techniques and guidelines, which we expect will allow surgeons and therapists to achieve the best possible outcomes in their practices. We hope that this issue serves as a vehicle to spread the forward steps made by world leading experts to surgeons and therapists in the field.

I am fortunate and indebted to my great friend, Dr. Steve Lee, in editing this issue. While my effort was directed toward assembling review on primary repair, Steve organized the review of the most difficult topics of secondary reconstruction. Over the last decade, a number of symposiums, or courses, in major congresses—the meetings of International Federation for Societies of Surgery of the Hand, Federation of European Societies for Surgery of the Hand, American Society for Surgery of the Hand, American Association for Surgery of the Hand, British Society for Surgery of the Hand, etc—have been dedicated to tendon repair compilations. You will find most of the contributors often are speakers and teachers of these courses. It is our goal to present a collection of their updated views and personal methods in this issue, which undoubtedly would enhance the educational mission in this field. In the list of contributors, you will find those masters who pioneered the current tendon repair methods, names that familiarly describe established surgical methods, or those whose work has greatly changed the way of our practice!

Hand Clin 29 (2013) xiii–xiv
http://dx.doi.org/10.1016/j.hcl.2013.03.004

Both of us are indebted to the contributors of this issue. They are true heroes in making this issue. Finally, we are obliged to acknowledge Yonah Korngold and Jennifer Flynn-Briggs, editors of Elsevier Inc, for their insight and assistance in the production of this issue.

Jin Bo Tang, MD
Affiliated Hospital of Nantong University
20 West Temple Road
Nantong, Jiangsu 226001, China

E-mail address:
jinbotang@yahoo.com

It is my distinct honor to co-edit this issue with one of the foremost experts in the field, Dr. Jin Bo Tang. My wife and I spent more than a week as guests of the unbelievably gracious Jin Bo and his lovely wife, Xiao Tian Wang. We traveled with other experts of tendon injuries: Robert Savage, Dan Mass, and Michael Sandow, spending time in Nantong, China, where Dr. Tang runs the hand surgery section with a large team of surgeons and researchers. Like many of us, Dr. Tang is continually striving to answer some of the questions that continue to plague us in our efforts to improve outcomes after tendon injuries in the hand. I am forever grateful for the friendship I have made with Jin Bo and my travel companions. I am equally grateful for all of the contributors to this issue. They range from my mentors, friends, and colleagues. We hope you enjoy this issue as we try to unravel the mysteries and challenges of improving how our patients do after treatment of these devastating and life-altering injuries.

Steve K. Lee, MD
Hospital for Special Surgery
535 East 70th Street
New York, NY 10021, USA

E-mail address:
steve.kichul.lee@gmail.com

Gliding Resistance and Modifications of Gliding Surface of Tendon
Clinical Perspectives

Peter C. Amadio, MD

KEYWORDS

• Gliding resistance • Friction • Lubrication • Adhesions • Rehabilitation

KEY POINTS

- The tendon surface in zone 2 is specially adapted for gliding; the lubricated surface forms a protective skinlike layer with a coefficient of friction similar to cartilage on cartilage, or ice on ice.
- Repair techniques that minimize friction have better results in animal models of tendon repair.
- Therapy that enables gliding yields better results in animal models and clinically.
- It is possible to modify the gliding surface to reduce friction through tissue engineering; such modifications result in fewer adhesions after tendon repair in animal models and, in some reports, clinically.
- Modification of the gliding surface of tendon grafts can convert an extrasynovial graft into the functional equivalent of an intrasynovial graft, with improved results in animal models.

The normal human digital flexor tendon in its sheath has a coefficient of friction similar to articular cartilage, which is maintained not only by synovial fluid lubrication but also by lubricants bound to the tendon surface, including hyaluronic acid, phospholipids, and a lubricating proteoglycan, lubricin. This system can be disrupted by degenerative conditions such as trigger finger, or by trauma. Restoration of a functioning gliding surface after injury can be helped by using low-friction, high-strength suture designs; therapy that enables gliding; and, at least experimentally, the addition of lubricants that can be fixed to the tendon surface covalently.[1] Such lubricants may be especially helpful when tendon grafts are needed, because the lubricants can significantly reduce the normal high friction of extrasynovial tendons,[1] which are the most common tendon graft donors.

The flexor tendon and digital sheath system is a marvel of nature's tissue engineering. The precise fit, lubrication, strength, motion, and mechanics are all designed to optimize efficiency, strength, and motion. This article reviews the relevant anatomy, mechanics, and biology, particularly as they affect the gliding surface.

NORMAL TENDON
Gliding Surface: The Tendon Skin

The tendon surface in the finger is specially adapted for gliding. The typical extrasynovial tendon is surrounded by an areolar paratenon (**Fig. 1**A),[2–5] which provides for good gliding, but, when this system is disrupted by injury, fibrosis and adhesions are the common result.[6,7] In contrast, the intrasynovial tendon has a different gliding system,

Commercial relationships: The author has a consulting contract with Holy Stone Healthcare Co, Ltd, Taipei, Taiwan.
Mayo Clinic, 200 First Street Southwest, Rochester, MN 55905, USA
E-mail address: pamadio@mayo.edu

Hand Clin 29 (2013) 159–166
http://dx.doi.org/10.1016/j.hcl.2013.02.001

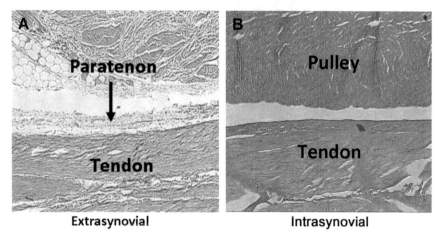

Fig. 1. (*A*) Typical extrasynovial tendon is surrounded by an areolar paratenon (×400). (*B*) intrasynovial tendon has no paratenon (×400).

with a coefficient of friction that is similar to articular cartilage,[8–11] and a gliding surface (see **Fig. 1**B) that includes the lubricating elements of hyaluronic acid, phospholipids, and a unique proteoglycan, lubricin.[10,12–14] This surface is durable, protecting the underlying collagen fibril network from abrasion after repetitive motion, not only in vivo but also in harsh in vitro conditions (**Fig. 2**).[15] This protective, low-friction surface serves as a barrier to tissue ingrowth, most likely as a result of the lubricin that is present, because lubricin is know to have anti–cell adhesion properties.[16–18] In many ways, the gliding surface of the flexor tendon in the digital sheath functions as a protective barrier, protecting the tendon much the way skin protects the organism.

Gliding Resistance

The gliding resistance of the tendon/pulley interface is affected by at least 3 factors: the coefficient of friction of the interface, which is normally very low; the load on the tendon; and the angle of the arc the tendon makes with the pulley.[19] The second and third factors combine to determine the perpendicular force between the tendon and pulley. The greater the angle of the arc of contact for a given tendon load, the greater the perpendicular force between tendon and pulley, and therefore the greater the frictional force. Mechanical principles emphasize that frictional force is not, in general, related to the size of the contact area, although the size and shape of the surface does play a role in fluid-lubricated situations, which is relevant to tendons, which are lubricated by synovial fluid within the tendon sheath.[10] Lubricants such as synovial fluid reduce friction between dry surfaces by separating the surfaces with a thin film of fluid, so that microscopic irregularities on the opposing surfaces do not touch one another. However, the motion of this lubricating fluid creates its own source of friction, called drag,

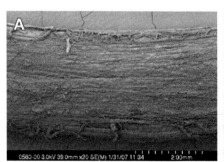
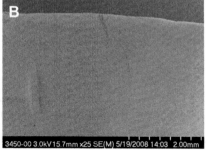

Fig. 2. (*A*) Extrasynovial surface after 1000 cycles of repetitive motion against a pulley (scanning electron microscope [SEM], ×20). (*B*) Intrasynovial surface after 1000 cycles of repetitive motion against a pulley (SEM, ×25).

which is related to the velocity of motion and the viscosity of the lubricant.[19] In total, the net effect of the boundary lubrication mechanism of tendon and pulley results in a coefficient of friction of around 0.02 to 0.03,[9,15] about the same as that between cartilage surfaces, and about an order of magnitude less than ice on ice.[20]

Differences Between Extrasynovial and Intrasynovial Tendons

As noted earlier, the gliding mechanisms of extrasynovial and intrasynovial tendons are different. The latter surface is optimized for gliding at low friction, and has a protective skin; the former does not. The result is obvious in repetitive loading testing, as noted in **Fig. 2**; the extrasynovial tendon abrades at a faster rate and becomes rougher under repetitive loads, which may explain, at least in part, the poor results of grafting using extrasynovial tendons to replace intrasynovial tendons clinically,[21–27] and in animal studies in vivo (**Fig. 3**).[5,7]

Differences Between Regions of Intrasynovial Tendons: Microenvironments

In addition to the differences between extrasynovial and intrasynovial tendons, there are also microenvironments within tendons that affect gliding ability. Most notably, within the tendon sheath are vincular vessels to the profundus and superficialis tendons, which may act as tethers to some extent. Most importantly, these vessels provide segmental vascular nutrition to the tendons,[28–30] and their integrity is important to tendon healing.[31]

TENDONS IN PATHOLOGIC CONDITIONS
Trigger Finger

The cause of trigger finger is not fully understood, but it is generally considered to be a degenerative condition of the flexor tendon, as also occurs in other species with intrasynovial tendons.[32,33] The tendon in trigger fingers may show microscopic calcification or other signs of degeneration.[34–37] Although the gliding resistance of trigger fingers is

unknown, the clinical presentation suggests that it must be increased. Lubricants have been used successfully to treat stenosing tenosynovitis in animals,[38] and has been suggested for humans as well.[39] However, the only available clinical study[39] compared steroid plus hyaluronate with surgery, with results in the nonsurgical group similar to those reported historically for trigger finger alone.[40–44]

Laceration

The gliding of tendons that have been lacerated is impaired, regardless of whether the laceration is complete[45] or partial,[46] or whether the injury is sutured[8] or, if partial, left unrepaired.[47] It is also clear from laboratory and clinical studies that both the gliding and healing of partially lacerated tendons (unless these are near complete) is better with trimming than with repair.[47,48]

EFFECTS OF TREATMENT ON TENDON GLIDING
Suture Type

The design of the tendon core suture is important to the ability of the tendon to glide. Low-profile repairs, such as the modified Kessler and its variants (**Fig. 4**A), have little suture material on the

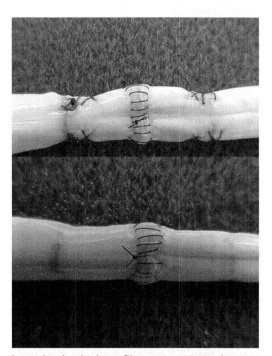

Fig. 4. (*Top*) A high-profile repair: MGH/Becker. Note exposed core suture on the palmar tendon surface. (*Bottom*) A low profile repair: modified Kessler. Note absence of exposed core suture on the palmar tendon surface.

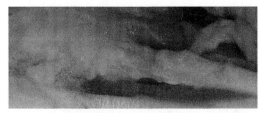

Fig. 3. Typical appearance of an extrasynovial tendon graft in a canine model in vivo after 6 weeks. Note extensive adhesions.

anterior tendon surface.[45,49–52] These repairs have low friction, and result in healing with fewer adhesions in animal models. In contrast, repairs with suture loops on the tendon surface, such as the MGH/Becker repair, have higher friction and result in more adhesions (see **Fig. 4**B). With regard to the epitendinous suture used to finish the repair in zone 2 injuries, all current designs have multiple loops on the tendon surface. Whether these loops are locked or not seems to have little impact on friction,[53] although one report did note increased resistance to the Lin technique of locking.[54] Because locking loops provide better gap resistance, these should be preferred, with the possible exception of the Lin method.[54]

Knot Location

The location of the knot is critically important to the amount of friction generated by a tendon repair. Knots on the tendon's anterior surface generate more friction than lateral knots, or knots inside the repair site.[52,55] Thus, for example, if the Tsuge repair is preferred, a double Tsuge method with the knots on the lateral tendon surface might be preferable to a more classic Tsuge repair, with the knots placed anteriorly.

Suture Materials

The suture material also has an effect on friction. Although it might be assumed that monofilament sutures have lower friction than braided sutures, the answer is more complex, because often monofilament sutures are made of different materials than braided ones, and braided sutures are more likely to have friction-lowering components such as polytetrafluoroethylene, polybutilate, or silicone included. In our tests, the suture material with the lowest friction has been braided polyester/monofilament polyethylene composite (FiberWire, Arthrex, Naples, FL).[56] However, these lower friction sutures also tend to hold a knot less well,[57] and the effect of suture material on the friction of the overall tendon repair is small.[56] In addition, although braided polyester/monofilament polyethylene composite sutures are stronger than some other commonly used materials, such as polypropylene, nylon, or braided polyester,[56,58] surgeons should be aware of size differences: for example, size 4-0 braided polyester/monofilament polyethylene composite has a greater cross-sectional diameter than 3-0 sutures made of other materials.[58] Thus, although suture materials vary in frictional coefficient, the effect of suture material on the overall friction of the suture construct is small, and surgeons should be aware of differences in cross section between sutures of nominally similar size.

TRIMMING OF PARTIALLY LACERATED TENDON

The surgical literature is clear that partially lacerated tendons heal better when trimmed than when sutured, unless the partial laceration is nearly complete.[59] Trimmed tendons also have less friction, and less tendency to trigger.[47] Thus, it has been my preference to trim partial lacerations and make a smooth divot in the tendon when the partial injury is less than 50% of the tendon diameter (**Fig. 5**). For larger injuries (up to 75%–90% lacerations; often it is difficult to accurately estimate the degree of partial injury visually, and so it may be better to err on the side of prudence and add a suture when in doubt), a running locked peripheral 6-0 finishing suture can be used. If the partial laceration is nearly complete, then I treat such injuries as complete lacerations.

Therapy

The effect of therapy on tendon gliding is related to the amount of loading that is applied to the tendon. Active motion programs ensure that the tendon is moving, but the load applied by the patient is difficult to control, and, if the load exceeds the holding power of the tendon suture (usually just a few kilograms in the early phases), the repair may break.[58,59] Passive motion and synergistic motion programs can provide more measured loads, but the familiar problem of trying to push a tendon through a pulley often limits gliding in the flexion direction.[60] Tanaka and colleagues[61] recently developed a modified synergistic method that provides some loading (roughly 100 g) in the proximal direction by maintaining metacarpophalangeal joint extension in both the flexion and extension phases of the synergistic program (**Fig. 6**). Place-and-hold methods are another way to provide a more gentle proximal pull on the tendon.[60,62]

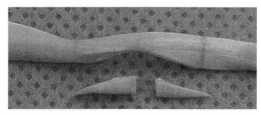

Fig. 5. Tendon trimming after partial tendon laceration.

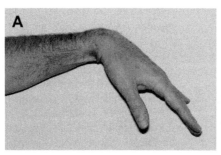 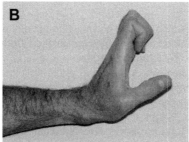

Fig. 6. Modified synergistic motion. (*A*) Wrist flexion phase, (*B*) wrist extension phase. (*Data from* Tanaka T, Amadio PC, Zhao C, et al. Flexor digitorum profundus tendon tension during finger manipulation. J Hand Ther 2005;18:330–8.)

Barriers

Mechanical adhesion barriers have been used for years in an attempt to improve the results of tendon repair.[38,63–71] However, although many agents have shown promise in animal models, few have proved to be reliably effective clinically.[72,73]

Hyaluronic Acid

Hyaluronic acid has been used as a barrier to adhesion formation for many years. Its use is based on the clinical observation that wounds bathed in synovial fluid often do not heal.[74] However, more recent studies suggest that the inhibitory effect is caused by another component of synovial fluid, lubricin.

Nonetheless, hyaluronic acid has been shown to be an effective barrier to adhesion formation in animal models, especially in highly cross-linked versions, which tend to have greater tissue resident time.[75] Methods are also available to fix cross-linked hyaluronic acid to the tendon surface with covalent bonds; such methods result in even longer residence time and, in animal models, reduced friction and fewer adhesions.[76] As suggested by the adhesion-inhibiting effect of lubricin, adding lubricin to the hyaluronic acid mixture results in even further adhesion prevention, although at the cost of increased rates of tendon rupture in animal models.[71]

Antimetabolites

The use of antimetabolites in tendon repair is has advantages and disadvantages. Unless they are highly targeted, drugs that reduce DNA or collagen synthesis not only block adhesions; they block healing. Beta-aminopropionitrile blocks collagen cross linking; it has been used experimentally to block adhesions since the 1960s, and is effective,[77] but because its potential side effects include aneurysm formation,[78] it has never engendered much enthusiasm with regard to clinical use.

The cancer chemotherapeutic agent 5-fluorouracil blocks DNA synthesis, and has a short duration of action when applied topically; it has been tried in tendon repair, and does reduce adhesions and improve tendon gliding,[79,80] but it may have a greater role in tenolysis, in which tendon integrity may be less of an issue.

THE FUTURE: TISSUE ENGINEERING OF THE GLIDING SURFACE

As noted earlier, the beneficial effects of hyaluronic acid on adhesion reduction and tendon lubrication can be extended by using 1-ethyl-3-(3-dimethylaminopropyl) carbodiimide to covalently bond carboxyl groups on hyaluronic acid molecules to amine groups on proteins on the tendon surface.[81,82] The addition of gelatin (denatured collagen) and N-hydroxysuccinimide improve the efficiency of the reaction.[82] With this treatment, the hyaluronic acid remains on the tendon surface for weeks rather than days.[76] We have used this reaction in our research to reduce the friction associated with both tendon repair and tendon grafting, in vitro and in vivo.[71,76,83,84] When lubricin is added, the results in terms of lubrication are even better, and a high friction extrasynovial tendon such as a palmaris longus can be provided with the coefficient of friction of an intrasynovial tendon such as the flexor profundus.[85]

In the future, it should be possible to improve the gliding and reduce the friction of human tendon repairs and, especially, tendon grafts, with such surface treatments. There could be a particular role for cases in which, because of other injuries (fracture, replantation, polytrauma), the patient is unable to participate in the usual early motion therapy program. In such cases, the use of attached surface lubricants may allow a delay in the initiating rehabilitation, while still minimizing adhesion formation. Our recently published preliminary data in an animal model show that this may be possible.[1]

SUMMARY

The smooth gliding of the normal human digital flexor is maintained not only by synovial fluid lubrication but also by lubricants bound to the tendon surface, including hyaluronic acid, phospholipids, and a lubricating proteoglycan, lubricin. This system can be disrupted by degenerative conditions such as trigger finger, or by trauma. The resistance to tendon gliding after surgical repair of the lacerated digital flexor tendon relates to location of suture knots, exposure of suture materials, and type of surgical repair and materials. Restoration of a functioning gliding surface after injury can be helped by using low-friction, high-strength suture designs; therapy that enables gliding; and, at least experimentally, the addition of lubricants that can be fixed to the tendon surface covalently. Such lubricants may be especially helpful when tendon grafts are needed, because the lubricants can significantly reduce the high friction of extrasynovial tendons.

REFERENCES

1. Zhao C, Sun YL, Jay GD, et al. Surface modification counteracts adverse effects associated with immobilization after flexor tendon repair. J Orthop Res 2012;30:1940–4.
2. Guimberteau JC. Endoscopic approach of the aponeurosis. Fibrillar continuity in fasciae and aponeurosis. Ann Chir Plast Esthet 2012;57:465–6 [in French].
3. Guimberteau JC, Delage JP, McGrouther DA, et al. The microvacuolar system: how connective tissue sliding works. J Hand Surg Eur 2010;35:614–22.
4. Guimberteau JC, Delage JP, Wong J, et al. The role and mechanical behavior of the connective tissue in tendon sliding. Chir Main 2010;29:155–66.
5. Guimberteau JC, Sentucq-Rigall J, Panconi B, et al. Introduction to the knowledge of subcutaneous sliding system in humans. Ann Chir Plast Esthet 2005;50:19–34 [in French].
6. Gelberman RH, Seiler JG 3rd, Rosenberg AE, et al. Intercalary flexor tendon grafts. A morphological study of intrasynovial and extrasynovial donor tendons. Scand J Plast Reconstr Surg Hand Surg 1992;26:257–64.
7. Abrahamsson SO, Gelberman R. Maintenance of the gliding surface of tendon autografts in dogs. Acta Orthop Scand 1994;65:548–52.
8. Coert JH, Uchiyama S, Amadio PC, et al. Flexor tendon-pulley interaction after tendon repair. A biomechanical study. J Hand Surg Br 1995;20:573–7.
9. Uchiyama S, Coert JH, Berglund L, et al. Method for the measurement of friction between tendon and pulley. J Orthop Res 1995;13:83–9.
10. Uchiyama S, Amadio PC, Ishikawa J, et al. Boundary lubrication between the tendon and the pulley in the finger. J Bone Joint Surg Am 1997;79: 213–8.
11. Uchiyama S, Amadio PC, Berglund LJ, et al. Analysis of the gliding pattern of the canine flexor digitorum profundus tendon through the A2 pulley. J Biomech 2008;41:1281–8.
12. Sun Y, Chen MY, Zhao C, et al. The effect of hyaluronidase, phospholipase, lipid solvent and trypsin on the lubrication of canine flexor digitorum profundus tendon. J Orthop Res 2008;26: 1225–9.
13. Sun Y, Berger EJ, Zhao C, et al. Mapping lubricin in canine musculoskeletal tissues. Connect Tissue Res 2006;47:215–21.
14. Sun Y, Berger EJ, Zhao C, et al. Expression and mapping of lubricin in canine flexor tendon. J Orthop Res 2006;24:1861–8.
15. Uchiyama S, Amadio PC, Coert JH, et al. Gliding resistance of extrasynovial and intrasynovial tendons through the A2 pulley. J Bone Joint Surg Am 1997;79:219–24.
16. Schaefer DB, Wendt D, Moretti M, et al. Lubricin reduces cartilage–cartilage integration. Biorheology 2004;41:503–8.
17. Rhee DK, Marcelino J, Baker M, et al. The secreted glycoprotein lubricin protects cartilage surfaces and inhibits synovial cell overgrowth. J Clin Invest 2005; 115:622–31.
18. Jay GD, Torres JR, Rhee DK, et al. Association between friction and wear in diarthrodial joints lacking lubricin. Arthritis Rheum 2007;56:3662–9.
19. An KN, Berglund L, Uchiyama S, et al. Measurement of friction between pulley and flexor tendon. Biomed Sci Instrum 1993;29:1–7.
20. Tanaka E, Kawai N, Tanaka M, et al. The frictional coefficient of the temporomandibular joint and its dependency on the magnitude and duration of joint loading. J Dent Res 2004;83:404–7.
21. Stark HH, Zemel NP, Boyes JH, et al. Flexor tendon graft through intact superficialis tendon. J Hand Surg Am 1977;2:456–61.
22. Forgon M, Biro V. Reconstruction of the digital tendon-sheath in "no-man's" land with autologous transplanted vein-graft. Hand 1978;10:28–36.
23. McClinton MA, Curtis RM, Wilgis EF. One hundred tendon grafts for isolated flexor digitorum profundus injuries. J Hand Surg Am 1982;7:224–9.
24. LaSalle WB, Strickland JW. An evaluation of the two-stage flexor tendon reconstruction technique. J Hand Surg Am 1983;8:263–7.
25. Strickland JW. Results of flexor tendon surgery in zone II. Hand Clin 1985;1:167–79.
26. Wehbe MA, Mawr B, Hunter JM, et al. Two-stage flexor-tendon reconstruction. Ten-year experience. J Bone Joint Surg Am 1986;68:752–63.

27. Amadio PC, Wood MB, Cooney WP 3rd, et al. Staged flexor tendon reconstruction in the fingers and hand. J Hand Surg Am 1988;13:559–62.

28. Leffert RD, Weiss C, Athanasoulis CA. The vincula; with particular reference to their vessels and nerves. J Bone Joint Surg Am 1974;56:1191–8.

29. Ochiai N, Matsui T, Miyaji N, et al. Vascular anatomy of flexor tendons. I. Vincular system and blood supply of the profundus tendon in the digital sheath. J Hand Surg Am 1979;4:321–30.

30. Manske PR, Lesker PA. Nutrient pathways of flexor tendons in primates. J Hand Surg Am 1982;7:436–44.

31. Amadio PC, Hunter JM, Jaeger SH, et al. The effect of vincular injury on the results of flexor tendon surgery in zone 2. J Hand Surg Am 1985;10:626–32.

32. Fortier LA, Nixon AJ, Ducharme NG, et al. Tenoscopic examination and proximal annular ligament desmotomy for treatment of equine "complex" digital sheath tenosynovitis. Vet Surg 1999;28:429–35.

33. Nixon AJ, Sams AE, Ducharme NG. Endoscopically assisted annular ligament release in horses. Vet Surg 1993;22:501–7.

34. Sampson SP, Badalamente MA, Hurst LC, et al. Pathobiology of the human A1 pulley in trigger finger. J Hand Surg Am 1991;16:714–21.

35. Sbernardori MC, Mazzarello V, Tranquilli-Leali P. Scanning electron microscopic findings of the gliding surface of the A1 pulley in trigger fingers and thumbs. J Hand Surg Eur 2007;32:384–7.

36. Drossos K, Remmelink M, Nagy N, et al. Correlations between clinical presentations of adult trigger digits and histologic aspects of the A1 pulley. J Hand Surg Am 2009;34:1429–35.

37. Gruber H, Peer S, Loizides A. The "dark tendon sign" (DTS): a sonographic indicator for idiopathic trigger finger. Ultrasound Med Biol 2011;37:688–92.

38. Gaughan EM, Nixon AJ, Krook LP, et al. Effects of sodium hyaluronate on tendon healing and adhesion formation in horses. Am J Vet Res 1991;52:764–73.

39. Callegari L, Spanò E, Bini A, et al. Ultrasound-guided injection of a corticosteroid and hyaluronic acid: a potential new approach to the treatment of trigger finger. Drugs R D 2011;11:137–45.

40. Sato ES, Gomes Dos Santos JB, Belloti JC, et al. Treatment of trigger finger: randomized clinical trial comparing the methods of corticosteroid injection, percutaneous release and open surgery. Rheumatology (Oxford) 2012;51:93–9.

41. Chambers RG Jr. Corticosteroid injections for trigger finger. Am Fam Physician 2009;80:454.

42. Peters-Veluthamaningal C, van der Windt DA, Winters JC, et al. Corticosteroid injection for trigger finger in adults. Cochrane Database Syst Rev 2009;(21):CD005617.

43. Benson LS, Ptaszek AJ. Injection versus surgery in the treatment of trigger finger. J Hand Surg Am 1997;22:138–44.

44. Buch-Jaeger N, Foucher G, Ehrler S, et al. The results of conservative management of trigger finger. A series of 169 patients. Ann Chir Main Memb Super 1992;11:189–93.

45. Moriya T, Zhao C, Yamashita T, et al. Effect of core suture technique and type on the gliding resistance during cyclic motion following flexor tendon repair: a cadaveric study. J Orthop Res 2010;28:1475–81.

46. Zhao C, Amadio PC, Zobitz ME, et al. Gliding resistance after repair of partially lacerated human flexor digitorum profundus tendon in vitro. Clin Biomech (Bristol, Avon) 2001;16:696–701.

47. Erhard L, Zobitz ME, Zhao C, et al. Treatment of partial lacerations in flexor tendons by trimming. A biomechanical in vitro study. J Bone Joint Surg Am 2002;84:1006–12.

48. Hajipour L, Gulihar A, Dias J. Effect of laceration and trimming of a tendon on the coefficient of friction along the A2 pulley: an in vitro study on turkey tendon. J Bone Joint Surg Br 2010;92:1171–5.

49. Tanaka T, Amadio PC, Zhao C, et al. Gliding characteristics and gap formation for locking and grasping tendon repairs: a biomechanical study in a human cadaver model. J Hand Surg Am 2004;29:6–14.

50. Paillard PJ, Amadio PC, Zhao C, et al. Gliding resistance after FDP and FDS tendon repair in zone II: an in vitro study. Acta Orthop Scand 2002;73:465–70.

51. Moriya T, Larson MC, Zhao C, et al. The effect of core suture flexor tendon repair techniques on gliding resistance during static cycle motion and load to failure: a human cadaver study. J Hand Surg Eur 2012;37:316–22.

52. Momose T, Amadio PC, Zhao C, et al. Suture techniques with high breaking strength and low gliding resistance: experiments in the dog flexor digitorum profundus tendon. Acta Orthop Scand 2001;72:635–41.

53. Moriya T, Zhao C, An KN, et al. The effect of epitendinous suture technique on gliding resistance during cyclic motion after flexor tendon repair: a cadaveric study. J Hand Surg Am 2010;35:552–8.

54. Kubota H, Aoki M, Pruitt DL, et al. Mechanical properties of various circumferential tendon suture techniques. J Hand Surg Br 1996;21:474–80.

55. Momose T, Amadio PC, Zhao C, et al. The effect of knot location, suture material, and suture size on the gliding resistance of flexor tendons. J Biomed Mater Res 2000;53:806–11.

56. Silva JM, Zhao C, An KN, et al. Gliding resistance and strength of composite sutures in human flexor digitorum profundus tendon repair: an in vitro biomechanical study. J Hand Surg Am 2009;34:87–92.

57. Abbi G, Espinoza L, Odell T, et al. Evaluation of 5 knots and 2 suture materials for arthroscopic rotator cuff repair: very strong sutures can still slip. Arthroscopy 2006;22:38–43.

58. Chesney A, Chauhan A, Kattan A, et al. Systematic review of flexor tendon rehabilitation protocols in zone II of the hand. Plast Reconstr Surg 2011;127: 1583–92.

59. Hung LK, Pang KW, Yeung PL, et al. Active mobilisation after flexor tendon repair: comparison of results following injuries in zone 2 and other zones. J Orthop Surg (Hong Kong) 2005;13:158–63.

60. Amadio PC. Friction of the gliding surface. Implications for tendon surgery and rehabilitation. J Hand Ther 2005;18:112–9.

61. Tanaka T, Amadio PC, Zhao C, et al. Flexor digitorum profundus tendon tension during finger manipulation. J Hand Ther 2005;18:330–8.

62. Trumble TE, Vedder NB, Seiler JG 3rd, et al. Zone-II flexor tendon repair: a randomized prospective trial of active place-and-hold therapy compared with passive motion therapy. J Bone Joint Surg Am 2010;92:1381–9.

63. Ferguson RE, Rinker B. The use of a hydrogel sealant on flexor tendon repairs to prevent adhesion formation. Ann Plast Surg 2006;56:54–8.

64. Meislin RJ, Wiseman DM, Alexander H, et al. A biomechanical study of tendon adhesion reduction using a biodegradable barrier in a rabbit model. J Appl Biomater 1990;1:13–9.

65. Mentzel M, Hoss H, Keppler P, et al. The effectiveness of ADCON-T/N, a new anti-adhesion barrier gel, in fresh divisions of the flexor tendons in Zone II. J Hand Surg Br 2000;25:590–2.

66. Rogers GJ, Milthorpe BK, Schindhelm K, et al. Shielding of augmented tendon–tendon repair. Biomaterials 1995;16:803–7.

67. Temiz A, Ozturk C, Bakunov A, et al. A new material for prevention of peritendinous fibrotic adhesions after tendon repair: oxidised regenerated cellulose (Interceed), an absorbable adhesion barrier. Int Orthop 2008;32:389–94.

68. McGonagle L, Jones MD, Dowson D, et al. The biotribological properties of anti-adhesive agents commonly used during tendon repair. J Orthop Res 2012;30:775–80.

69. Moro-oka T, Miura H, Mawatari T, et al. Mixture of hyaluronic acid and phospholipid prevents adhesion formation on the injured flexor tendon in rabbits. J Orthop Res 2000;18:835–40.

70. Stark HH, Boyes JH, Johnson L, et al. The use of paratenon, polyethylene film, or silastic sheeting to prevent restricting adhesions to tendons in the hand. J Bone Joint Surg Am 1977;59:908–13.

71. Zhao C, Sun YL, Kirk RL, et al. Effects of a lubricin-containing compound on the results of flexor tendon repair in a canine model in vivo. J Bone Joint Surg Am 2010;92:1453–61.

72. Golash A, Kay A, Warner JG, et al. Efficacy of ADCON-T/N after primary flexor tendon repair in Zone II: a controlled clinical trial. J Hand Surg Br 2003;28:113–5.

73. Riccio M, Battiston B, Pajardi G, et al. Efficiency of Hyaloglide in the prevention of the recurrence of adhesions after tenolysis of flexor tendons in zone II: a randomized, controlled, multicentre clinical trial. J Hand Surg Eur 2010;35:130–8.

74. Andrish J, Holmes R. Effects of synovial fluid on fibroblasts in tissue culture. Clin Orthop Relat Res 1979;(138):279–83.

75. Pitarresi G, Palumbo FS, Calabrese R, et al. Cross-linked hyaluronan with a protein-like polymer: novel bioresorbable films for biomedical applications. J Biomed Mater Res A 2008;84:413–24.

76. Zhao C, Sun YL, Amadio PC, et al. Surface treatment of flexor tendon autografts with carbodiimide-derivatized hyaluronic acid. An in vivo canine model. J Bone Joint Surg Am 2006;88:2181–91.

77. Peacock EE Jr, Madden JW. Some studies on the effects of beta-aminopropionitrile in patients with injured flexor tendons. Surgery 1969;66:215–23.

78. Kanematsu Y, Kanematsu M, Kurihara C, et al. Pharmacologically induced thoracic and abdominal aortic aneurysms in mice. Hypertension 2010;55: 1267–74.

79. Moran SL, Ryan CK, Orlando GS, et al. Effects of 5-fluorouracil on flexor tendon repair. J Hand Surg Am 2000;25:242–51.

80. Zhao C, Zobitz ME, Sun YL, et al. Surface treatment with 5-fluorouracil after flexor tendon repair in a canine in vivo model. J Bone Joint Surg Am 2009;91:2673–82.

81. Momose T, Amadio PC, Sun YL, et al. Surface modification of extrasynovial tendon by chemically modified hyaluronic acid coating. J Biomed Mater Res 2002;59:219–24.

82. Sun YL, Yang C, Amadio PC, et al. Reducing friction by chemically modifying the surface of extrasynovial tendon grafts. J Orthop Res 2004;22:984–9.

83. Tanaka T, Sun YL, Zhao C, et al. Optimization of surface modifications of extrasynovial tendon to improve its gliding ability in a canine model in vitro. J Orthop Res 2006;24:1555–61.

84. Zhao C, Sun YL, Ikeda J, et al. Improvement of flexor tendon reconstruction with carbodiimide-derivatized hyaluronic acid and gelatin-modified intrasynovial allografts: study of a primary repair failure model. J Bone Joint Surg Am 2010;92:2817–28.

85. Taguchi M, Zhao C, Sun YL, et al. The effect of surface treatment using hyaluronic acid and lubricin on the gliding resistance of human extrasynovial tendons in vitro. J Hand Surg Am 2009;34:1276–81.

Tendon Healing, Edema, and Resistance to Flexor Tendon Gliding: Clinical Implications

Ya Fang Wu, MD, Jin Bo Tang, MD*

KEYWORDS

- Tendon healing • Tenocyte proliferation • Apoptosis • Adhesions • Resistance to tendon gliding
- Edema • Annular pulleys • Early mobilization

KEY POINTS

- Early flexor tendon healing is characterized by peak cellular apoptosis of cells in the tendons in the first week, followed by progressively greater tenocyte proliferation in the second and third weeks.
- Apoptosis is a predominant event of the tenocytes in the middle and late healing periods, contributing to remodeling and restoration of tendon gliding surface. Tenocyte proliferation is minimal in these periods.
- Edema in subcutaneous tissue and the tendon is an inevitable biologic process, adding substantially to the resistance to tendon gliding. Major annular pulleys may greatly resist gliding of a repaired and swelling tendon.
- Experimentally, edema of the subcutaneous tissues contributed 20% to 25%, the intact A2 pulley 30%, and extensor tendons 15% to 20% of total resistance to the gliding of the flexor tendon. Tendon bulkiness (swelling and surgical repairs) also greatly contributes to the resistance.
- The contribution made by each of the factors changes dynamically with timing elapsed since surgery and the position of finger flexion. The overall resistance to tendon motion is progressively increased when the digit is extremely flexed.

The difficulties in functional recovery after digital flexor tendon injury stem from the weak healing capability of the tendon itself. Although the tendon has healing capacity through proliferation and collagen synthesis by tenocytes, the healing process is slow and usually weak in the first few weeks. This process causes 2 major problems—repair rupture and adhesion formation. During early tendon mobilization after surgery, repair rupture is the result of weak tendon healing as well as increases in resistance to tendon motion. Additionally, adhesions form because of insufficient tendon gliding. During the early tendon healing period, another factor also exerts a great influence on resistance to tendon gliding—edema formation, an inevitable biologic process after surgery to subcutaneous tissues and the tendon itself. Edema peaks a few days after surgery and persists as long as biologic healing processes are active.

Tendon healing, edema, resistance to tendon gliding, and formation of adhesions around the tendon are all innately associated. Their intricate relationship has become clearer over the past decade, and elucidation of their relationship has brought about modifications in surgical and postsurgical treatment of the digital flexor tendons.

Financial Disclosure: Supported by the grants from National Science Foundation of China (81030035 and 81271985) and Health Bureau of Jiangsu Province, Jiangsu, China.
Department of Hand Surgery, The Hand Surgery Research Center, Affiliated Hospital of Nantong University, 20 West Temple Road, Nantong, Jiangsu 226001, China
* Corresponding author.
E-mail address: jinbotang@yahoo.com

Hand Clin 29 (2013) 167–178
http://dx.doi.org/10.1016/j.hcl.2013.02.002
0749-0712/13/$ – see front matter © 2013 Elsevier Inc. All rights reserved.

hand.theclinics.com

TENDON HEALING

Tenocytes were once believed incapable of proliferating and repairing the lacerated tendon, and tendon healing was thought to rely on the invasion of peripheral cells and blood vessels, which frequently lead to formation of restrictive adhesions.[1,2] However, this concept was challenged in the 1970s and 80s. A large body of biologic and molecular evidence confirmed that tenocytes actively participate in tissue repair and that tendons are capable of healing from injury and revitalizing themselves. This process is dominated by tenocyte proliferation and production of their surrounding extracellular matrix early after surgical repair and by tendon surface remodeling and collagen realignment in the late healing stage.[3,4] How the tenocyte proliferation is balanced with other cellular events during the early tendon healing period and how tenocytes are cleared after tendon healing is complete have been partly elucidated by recent studies.[5–11]

Early Healing Stage: Peak Apoptosis Followed by Gradual Proliferation of Tenocytes

After tissue injury, cellular apoptosis and proliferation are closely associated and elegantly balanced through the entire healing period.[5–8] In a rat central 1/3 patellar tendon injury model,[8] apoptosis of the healing tendon was found to increase on day 14 and reached a maximum on day 28 after injury. However, proliferative cells reached a maximum population at day 4 and remained high up to day 28. Afterward, the number of both apoptotic and proliferative cells reduced and gradually returned to normal levels. We studied cellular apoptosis and proliferation of the repaired digital flexor tendon in a chicken model.[9] The tendons were stained with an in situ terminal deoxynucleotidyl transferase dUTP nick end labeling (TUNEL) assay to detect apoptotic cells over a 12-week period after surgical repair. We also stained the proliferating cell nuclear antigen (PCNA) and Bcl-2 (an antiapoptotic protein) to assess responses suppressive to cell apoptosis.

In uninjured tendons, only 3% ± 2% of the tenocytes showed signs of apoptosis and 1% ± 1% showed signs of active proliferation. The percentage of apoptotic cells went up to more than 40% at days 3 to 7 after tendon injury; on day 3, the number of inflammatory cells in the wound site also peaked. The number of TUNEL-positive cells, presumably composed mainly of inflammatory cells as well as tenocytes, peaked during the very early days in the healing process (days 3 and 7 in our chicken model).

In contrast, the number of PCNA-positive cells did not significantly increase until day 7 and peaked during days 7 to 21. At day 28, the number of PCNA-positive cells dropped; Bcl-2–positive cells showed parallel changes. We found that tenocyte apoptosis is typically accelerated within several days after injury, followed by increases in proliferation of tenocytes in 2 to 4 weeks with activation of molecular events to inhibit apoptosis (**Fig. 1**).

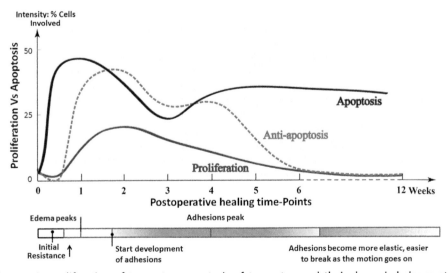

Fig. 1. Changes in proliferation of tenocytes, apoptosis of tenocytes, and their dynamic balance at different tendon healing periods. In the initial days after trauma and surgery, apoptosis peaks and proliferation declines, but from week 2 to 3, proliferation peaks and apoptosis declines. After week 4, apoptosis dominates while proliferation is minimal. Associated changes in edema and formation of adhesions are shown as well.

Middle and Late Healing Stages: Persistent Apoptosis with Greatly Declined Proliferation of Tenocytes

In the next step of our in vivo studies, we quantified cell apoptosis and proliferation during the middle and late healing stages.[10] We recorded cell apoptosis separately at the junction site of the repair and away from the junction site (ie, the extended regions), as well as regions of surface and core. The percentage of apoptotic tenocytes was generally higher on the surface of the tendon compared with that in the core, indicating a greater need for cellular clearance and surface remodeling in the surface region in the middle to late periods.

We recorded that the total cell population did not start to decline until after day 56 (2 months). Cell apoptosis persisted at a relatively high level on the tendon surface even at 3 months. Cell apoptosis in the core region declined after 2 months. These findings indicate that active tendon remodeling persists through the very late tendon healing period, especially on the tendon surface. In sharp contrast to tenocyte apoptosis, proliferation of tenocytes declined drastically after week 4, with less than 5% of the PCNA-positive cells in the tendon. At weeks 8 to 12, PCNA-positive cells returned to nearly normal levels. This finding points to the fact that in the middle and late tendon healing periods tenocyte apoptosis is a dominant event; it may even be a major biologic event in the remodeling and restoration of the gliding surface.

The percentage of apoptotic tenocytes ranged between 30% and 40% in the total cell population in both surface and core regions in the middle and late healing periods, except at the junction regions at week 8 (around 45%). Tenocyte apoptosis was slightly greater in the junction sites of the surgical repair, but generally apoptotic tenocytes did not exceed 40%; this indicates that apoptosis is at a relatively high level in the middle and late periods, but is still lower than in the first few days after surgery.

In areas distant from the junction site, apoptosis is more prominent in the tendon surface than in the tendon core. The increase in cellular apoptosis in the surface region is likely associated with the clearance of excess cells, which serves to promote formation of smooth gliding surfaces by remodeling adhesions. The junction region encompasses the greatest cellularity and the most robust healing reactions. Clearance of cells and reestablishment of collagenous connection can be a major event in the junction site in the late healing period.

Cellular Apoptosis in Adhesions

We then extended our investigation to adhesions forming around the repaired flexor tendons after a complete cut and surgical repair of the digital flexor tendon and 3 weeks of immobilization of the chicken toes. We correlated tendon gliding excursions recorded with a tensile testing machine as well as adhesion severity scores with degrees of cellular apoptosis. The percentage of apoptotic cells was noted to increase from the tendon core, to the tendon surface and to the adhesion-tendon interface, with that in the adhesion core the highest. The percentages of apoptotic cells in adhesions and at the adhesion-tendon gliding interface were generally 50% to 65%. The percentage of apoptotic cells was as high as 69% in the adhesion over the junction site of the tendon ends. Analysis of apoptotic index (ie, the percentage of apoptotic cells) against tendon excursions and severity of adhesions indicates that the tendons with more severe adhesions, or a lower excursion, see greater apoptosis in their adhesions and adhesion-tendon interfaces (**Fig. 2**).

Cellular apoptosis in the adhesions and at the adhesion-tendon interface may contribute to the fate of adhesions and the restoration of tendon gliding surface. This suggestion is consistent with the results of Wong and colleagues,[11] who reported that more apoptotic reactions were generally observed in the subcutaneous tissue and the immediate vicinity of the tendon toward the end of tendon healing in a mouse tendon injury model. We believe that the increases in cellular apoptosis at the adhesion and the tendon-adhesion interface are associated with the effect of shear deformation induced by mobilization. More apoptosis of cells in the tendon-adhesion interface would accelerate the recovery of the smooth gliding surface.

Microdynamics of Adhesions at Different Stages of Tendon Healing

The mechanical characteristics of adhesion tissues determine tendon gliding, but this relationship has rarely been investigated. We performed an in vivo study to determine the microdynamic features of adhesions in the middle and late healing period (postoperative weeks 4–8). The tendon with surrounding adhesions was harvested en bloc. A 1-cm tendon segment centered on the cut site was excised dorsally, but the adhesions medial, lateral and palmar to the tendon were kept intact, which bridged the 2 tendon stumps (**Fig. 3**), leaving the tendon ends connected solely by adhesions. The samples were then subjected to cyclic loading tests at 2, 5, 10, and 15 N for 10 cycles each.

The adhesions harvested at week 4 were the strongest, which survived at loads of 2 and 5 N and disrupted at 10 or 15 N. In contrast, adhesions at week 6 disrupted at loads of 5 or 10 N, although

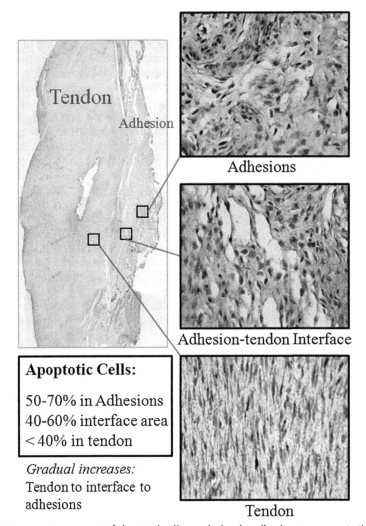

Fig. 2. Fifty percent to seventy percent of the total cell population in adhesions are apoptotic. The next highest proportion of apoptotic cells is seen in the tendon-adhesion gliding interface (40%–60%), and the fewest apoptotic cells are seen in the tendon core (<40%). Apoptosis is a predominant finding in the late healing stage.

all withstood a 2-N load. The failure load of the adhesions at week 8 was the lowest, from 2 to 5 N. We recorded minimal plastic deformation of the adhesion at week 4 (an average of 0.5 mm/N) and moderately large deformation at week 6 (1.3 mm/N) after cyclic loading at 2 N for 10 cycles (see **Fig. 3**). At week 8, the plastic deformity was the greatest. This biomechanical test revealed that the plasticity and strength of adhesions vary substantially in the course of tendon healing—the ability of adhesion tissues to resist tension decreases and tissue flexibility increases from middle to late healing stages. The microdynamic features of adhesion tissues determine the sliding amplitude of the tendon and how the tendon responds to postoperative motion.

Microdynamic features of adhesions and tenocytes apoptosis are associated—as apoptosis of cells in the adhesions goes on, the adhesions are more easily broken up after the adhesions are loaded. Digital motion would certainly reduce the strength and increase the elasticity of the adhesion fibers. We assume that the external force applied to move the tendon during digital motion, transferred to shear force over the adhesions and adhesion-tendon gliding interface, acts to continuously stimulate cellular apoptosis, in turn reducing the density and strength of the adhesion fibers, resulting in an increasingly greater elasticity and breakup of the adhesion fibers in the late healing stage (see **Fig. 3**).

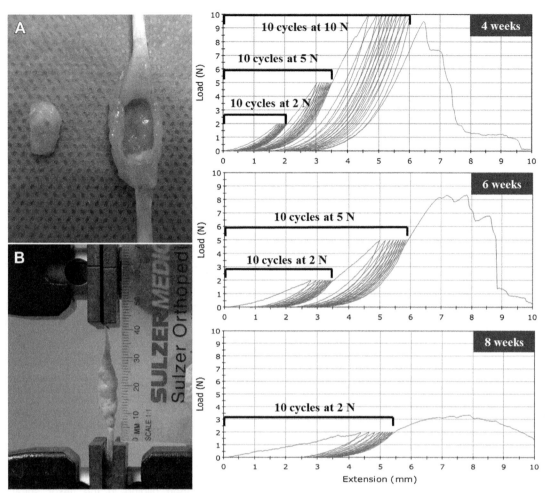

Fig. 3. The test method of microdynamic features of the adhesions. (*A*) Removal of a segment of tendon centered by the repair site and dorsal adhesions from the dorsal aspect of the tendon. (*B*) Test of breaking strengths and elasticity of the adhesions connecting the tendon. The right 3 graphs show how the adhesions harvested at 4, 6, and 8 weeks survived under different loads. The microdynamic features relate to how the adhesions resist tendon gliding and how easily these adhesions can be broken because of tensile load during active tendon gliding. The adhesions are more resistant to force in the midperiod of the healing than in the late period, indicating that a persistent mobilization of the digits up to the late healing stage is very important to fully restore tendon function.

Molecular Therapies to Reduce Adhesion Formation

Previous studies showed that expression of transforming growth factor (TGF)-β1 is upregulated in the early tendon healing period,[12–14] which is considered to be responsible for the formation of scars such as adhesions around healing digital flexor tendons. We also found in the lacerated digital flexor tendons of the chicken substantial upregulation of the TGF-β1, in contrast to little (or no) increase in platelet-derived growth factor and vascular endothelial growth factor and downregulation of the basic fibroblast growth factor gene expression.[14] Use of antibodies to neutralize

TGF-β1 has been shown to increase range of digital motion.[15] Gene therapy approaches to deliver synthesized small interfering RNA or microRNA (miRNA) to regulate the level of gene expression offers novel therapeutic potentials for a variety of pathologic conditions.[16] We designed the engineered miRNA and delivered the engineered miRNA to silence expression of the TGF-β1gene.[17]

Engineered miRNA was shown to downregulate TGF-β expression in vitro and in vivo.[17] The functional evaluation of this gene modulation approach is under way in our group. We also intended to use nanoparticles loaded with miRNAs to inhibit TGF-β1 gene expression to reduce the adhesions. This study is also ongoing in our lab.

Improving tendon healing strength through molecular modulation has been attempted and proved difficult, with varying results in animal models.[18–21] Currently, a few growth factors have been shown to enhance tendon healing strength, but their effectiveness appears to depend greatly on the persistence of expression of exogenous growth factors and the methods of delivery to the tendons. We expect to see more exciting results in future years in the molecular regulation of tendon healing.

EDEMA FORMATION AFTER TENDON REPAIR
Subcutaneous Tissue Edema: in vitro and in vivo Studies

Edema of both peritendinous tissues and tendons inevitably persists in the early period of tendon healing. Our group tried to characterize how the extent of peritendinous edema affects the amount of energy required for digital flexion and force of tendon gliding during simulated active digital motion.[22] Edema in subcutaneous tissue was reproduced in vitro in 3 different severities (mild, moderate, and severe) and 3 lengths (1 cm, 2 cm, and 3 cm) along the chicken toes.

Subcutaneous tissue edema was found to increase energy and force required to move the tendons. Increases in the severity of edema produced 2-fold or 3-fold greater resistance to tendon gliding, but changes in the length of the edematous tissue increased the resistance by only 10% to 30% in the presence of mild, moderate or severe edema (**Fig. 4**).[22] In other words, the resistance to tendon gliding was affected more by the severity of tissue edema than by the extension of edema in the digits, which suggests that edema severity is a concern in determining the timing of commencement and methods of tendon motion exercise.

Our continuing in vivo studies validated the in vitro findings. Through measuring edema in the chicken toes over a 2-week period after surgery involving tendon cut and repair,[23] we noted that the resistance to motion of the repaired tendon increased progressively for the first 4 days and remained consistent from days 4 to 7. More severe edema corresponded to greater tendon gliding force and work of digital flexion on each of the initial 5 post surgical days. We therefore suggested that the opportune time to start digital motion is from the fourth to seventh day after surgery to avoid overlapping the period of increased resistance. We also noted that repetitive motion of the digit over a number of cycles (6 in this study) greatly reduced the force and energy of the digital flexion. We suggested passive motion, intended to eliminate finger stiffness, as a "warm-up" measure before more aggressive active digital flexion.[23]

Xie and colleagues,[24] Halikis and colleagues,[25] and Zhao and colleagues[26,27] have also reported the force and energy required to move the tendon in the initial days after surgery in animal models. Most findings support a later start (3–5 days delay) of postoperative motion to avoid the period of increasing resistance presumably from postoperative edema.

Edema Inevitably Presents in the Repaired Tendons

Edema of the tendon is a common finding during delayed primary repair and is especially detrimental to tendon gliding in the flexor sheath region, as the swelling takes up room inside the narrow tendon gliding tunnel. Edema of the tendon increases resistance to tendon gliding, and many surgeons have found that repair of both superficialis and profundus tendons is particularly difficult in the delayed primary repair. Clinically, the senior

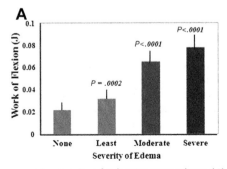
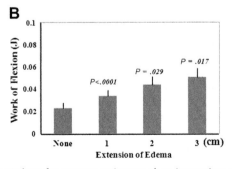

Fig. 4. Increases in severity of subcutaneous edema (A) produce far greater resistance than increasing extension of edema (B). Data and P values are obtained from 22 chicken toes after creation of different severity or extension of edema, respectively. These findings indicate that severity of edema, clinically judged by increases in diameter of the digits, loss of skin folds, etc., are more influential to the resistance; whether the edema is localized or extended in the hand is less influential.

author (JBT) often finds it hard to repair the superficialis tendon if the repair is delayed for 1 to 2 weeks. Tight closure of the sheath is harmful to the gliding of the edematous tendons.

Earlier experimental studies by our group support an opening (or nonrepair) of the damaged digital sheath, and partial venting of the annular pulleys if necessary, to accommodate the edematous tendons.[28,29] This policy is particularly relevant in delayed primary repair. In primary flexor tendon repair, the tendons do not swell at the time of surgery but do become edematous a few days later. This swelling contributes to the resistance to tendon gliding during early postoperative motion. From a few days to a few weeks after surgery, the repaired tendon at the repair site always has a greater diameter than a normal tendon, which is an important consideration in planning both surgery and rehabilitation.

Self-adhesive tapes could produce energy of digital flexion 4 times the baseline values.[30] Removal of dressing decreases the resistance to tendon motion.

Edema Peaks in the First Week and Persists in the Later Weeks; Adhesions Start to Form in the Second Week

Mobilization regimes initiated days after tendon repair are intended to prevent adhesion formation and joint stiffness. In the chicken tendon cut-and-repair model, we found no adhesion formation within the first 7 days after surgery.[31] Granulation tissue or filmy adhesions were seen at day 9, but no well-formed adhesions around the tendons were detected. At day 14, loose adhesions were found around the repaired tendons, which to some degree were restrictive to tendon gliding. The gliding force and energy required to move the tendon increased progressively from day 0 to day 3, but did not increase between days 3 and 9.[31]

We found that the early postoperative changes have 3 stages: *initial* (days 0–3, increasing resistance with development of edema), *delayed* (days 4–7, higher but consistent resistance with continuing edema), and *late* (after day 7–9, hardening of subcutaneous tissue with development of adhesions) (**Box 1**, see **Fig. 1**).[31] Based on these findings and the stage classification, we suggest that mobilization be delayed to avoid most of the period of increased resistance to mobilization of the injured tendons, possibly not starting until 4 or 5 days after repair. Digital motion may be started as late as day 7 or 9 for patients who are unable to start earlier. Adhesions do not form before then, and motion in the initial few days

---

> **Box 1**
> **Edema within 2 weeks post-repair and severity scores**
>
> *Major changes of edema and resistance to the tendon[31]*
>
> *Days 0–3*: increasing resistance with development of edema
>
> *Days 4–7, 9*: consistent resistance with continuing edema
>
> *Days 7, 9–14*: hardening of edematous tissues; adhesions start
>
> *Cao and Tang edema severity score[23] for recording the degree of edema:*
>
> 0 (none): swelling is absent
>
> 1 (slight): swelling is minimal or slight
>
> 2 (moderate): swelling is prominent with increases in digital diameter
>
> 3 (severe): swelling with opening in skin incision

---

may not affect recovery, but would only increase the pain of patients and workload of therapists.

RESISTANCE TO FLEXOR TENDON GLIDING

Resistance to tendon gliding is an important consideration, as ideally postoperative tendon motion should counteract all forces resisting digital motion without rupturing the repaired tendon. The following 10 factors are a list of factors in resistance to tendon gliding: (1) surgical repairs, (2) tendon bulkiness (tendon edema and bulkiness produced by surgical repair), (3) smoothness of tendon gliding surface, (4) healing responses of the tendons, (5) presence of intact constructive annular pulleys, (6) edema formation, (7) adhesion formation, (8) joint stiffness, (9) extensor tendon tethering, and (10) splints and bandages, and speed, frequency, and methods of postoperative motion. All these factors should be considered in designing a motion protocol and in instructing patients to follow a protocol. The protocol should be fine-tuned to counterbalance the increases in resistance to tendon motion when used in individual patients.

How edema and adhesions contribute to the resistance to tendon gliding is discussed ealier. Therefore, here the authors discuss how the presence of the flexor digitorum superficialis (FDS) tendon, major annular pulleys, the extensors, and joint stiffness contribute to the resistance to tendon gliding. Each type of surgical repair may contribute to gliding resistance of the tendon differently; many previous papers[32–35] have discussed this subject, so will not be discussed here.

Resistance Caused by Repaired Flexor Superficialis Tendons

Removal of one slip of the FDS tendon decreases the gliding resistance after flexor digitorum profundus (FDP) repair.[36] In cadaveric fingers,[37] we found that after incision of the FDS tendon proximal to, under, and distal to the A2 pulley, work of digital flexion of the intact FDP tendon decreased by 6%, 18%, and 20%, respectively, when compared with that with the FDS intact. Removal of the FDS under the A2 pulley affected the gliding of the FDP most manifestly. Removal of the FDS proximal to the A2 pulley had a less notable effect, and removal of the FDS distally did not alter the biomechanics of the FDP tendon substantially.

In a chicken tendon cut-and-repair model, we found that excision of the FDS tendon decreased resistance to FDP tendon gliding.[38] At the end of the eighth week, the excursions and work of digital flexion were better with the FDS excised than those with both tendon repairs when the tendons were cut within the pulley, and adhesions were more severe when both tendons were repaired. Those findings suggest that repairs of both FDS and FDP tendons in the area of the A2 pulley carry the risk of worsening the FDP tendon gliding. The repaired FDS, FDP, and intact A2 pulley may get stuck in some cases, allowing little tendon motion. We thus consider that if tendon injury is unclean, or tendon repair is delayed, repair of the FDS tendon together with FDP tendon may not be a wise decision. Either the FDS can be left unrepaired (or excised locally), the A2 pulley can be sufficiently vented, or both.

Resistance Caused by an Intact A2 Pulley

Segmentally located annular pulleys are one of the defining features of the digital flexor tendon system. These pulleys play important roles in keeping the tendon close to the joint rotation axis during finger flexion, preventing tendon bowstringing. However, such a biomechanical advantage comes at the cost of a strict limitation of gliding space within the sheath tunnel, in particular at the sites covered by the pulleys. Movement of a normal tendon is smooth; flexor pulleys and the tendons are an elegantly coordinated press-fit system. Nevertheless, the swelling and biologic healing responses of lacerated tendons disturb this system, hindering the gliding of swollen tendons. Resistance increases when the tendon repair site is located underneath the pulleys. The A2 pulley is the longest pulley in the digits, presenting a major hindrance to tendon motion in such cases.

Over the past decade, an increasing number of surgeons have sought to judiciously vent a part of the A2 pulley to "free" the repaired tendon, and this has been a major paradigm shift in treatment of the major pulley during flexor tendon repair (**Fig. 5**).[39–43] Pulley venting during repair is intended to facilitate tendon exposure, permit smoother tendon gliding without catching on the rim of the pulley edge, make room for postoperative tendon edema, and prevent postoperative tendon entrapment by adhesions.

Previous mechanical results support venting the A2 pulley up to 50% in cadaver studies.[44–46] In an in vivo model, we found that incision of the pulley improved excursion of the FDP tendon and decreased the work of digital flexion.[47] We also noted that rupture rates of the repaired tendons were greater in the toes with an intact A2 pulley compared with those with the pulley venting at postoperative weeks 2 and 4.[48] Venting of the pulley alters the force distribution in the tendon under the rigid pulley. In fact, in a subsequent study repair strength in lacerated FDP tendons was found to increase if the A2 pulley was vented.[49]

The relative contributions of tissue edema, tendon edema, and the intact A2 pulley to resistance to tendon gliding have been studied as well.[50] At postoperative weeks 1 and 2, work of digital flexion decreased by 19% to 25% with removal of the volar 2 cm soft tissues and further

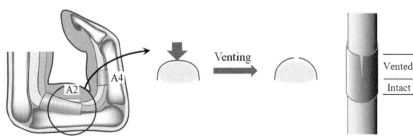

Fig. 5. Venting major pulleys reduces constriction to the tendon and reduces the chances of impingement of the repair site to the pulley rims. The A2 pulley can be vented to 1/2 to 2/3 of its length; a portion of this pulley is kept.

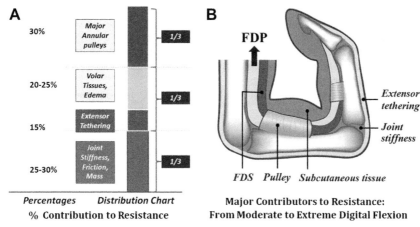

Fig. 6. (*A*) Percentage contribution of different factors to resistance to tendon motion. (*B*) Structures causing resistance to tendon gliding. Note that some factors can be eliminated *during surgery*: restrictive pulleys constitute about 30% of the total resistance, so venting of the constrictive portions of pulleys would decrease the resistance. Influences from other factors, such as extensor tethering or joint stiffness (contributing 30%–35% of total resistance), can be reduced by *repeated passive digital motion* before active tendon motion.

decreased by 30% to 34% with division of the A2 pulley. In other words, presence of an intact A2 pulley adds greater resistance than volar edematous subcutaneous tissue.

Effect of Joint Stiffness and Extensor Tethering

Little has been published regarding the effect of joint stiffness and extensor tethering on tendon gliding after surgery. Although these 2 factors have no direct bearing on tendon surgery, they do contribute to tendon gliding resistance. In a chicken model, we sequentially removed the volar subcutaneous tissue, extensor tendons, and flexor pulleys to try to understand the relative contribution of each of these surrounding tissues to tendon gliding resistance. Constrictive pulleys accounted for about 30% of all the resistance to digital flexion when the FDP tendon was injured; the subcutaneous tissue 10% to 25% (about 10% in normal toe and 20%–25% in injured FDP tendon); the FDS tendon about 10%; and the remaining portion (35%) should come from the combined effects of extensor tethering, joint stiffness, and mass of the digit (**Fig. 6**).

Finally, we must emphasize that finger joints are inherently small, and development of stiffness is frequent. At any phase along the flexion arc, if stiffness of these joints presents an obstacle to active tendon movement, the entire scale of contributing factors would be changed. Joint stiffness would become the overwhelmingly major resistance to tendon gliding. Each factor's contribution to the resistance of tendon gliding is a dynamic process, which varies depending on joint position, relative

position of the tendon repair site to the pulleys, and preconditioning of the tendon and adhesion tissues.

The overall resistance to tendon motion is progressively increased when the digit is extremely flexed (**Fig. 7**). Extreme active flexion of the fingers would (1) cause the impingement of repair sites to the sheath or pulley rims, (2) increase the bulkiness

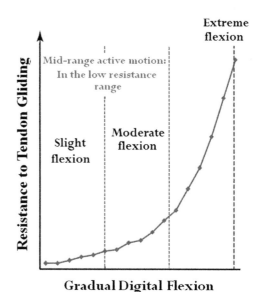

Fig. 7. The active digital motion creates a dynamic loading situation in which tendons are consistently subjected to changing forces from digital extension to flexion. Extreme flexion of the fingers greatly increases resistance to flexor tendon gliding. Therefore, in the early postoperative period, midrange active motion is in the low-resistance range and is preferable.

of tendon, (3) narrow the tendon gliding tunnel, (4) increase the tethering of the extensor mechanism, (5) tighten the capsule of the digital joints, and (6) increase the compression of edematous subcutaneous tissues. In the early postoperative period, midrange active motion is in the low-resistance range and is preferable in active motion of the fingers.

Therefore, to maximize functional recovery it is important to take all these factors into consideration when judging the dynamic relationship in designing individualized motion protocols.

SUMMARY

Early flexor tendon healing is characterized by peak cellular apoptosis of both inflammatory and tendon cells in the first week, followed by progressively greater tenocyte proliferation in the second and third weeks. Tenocyte apoptosis is a predominant event in the middle and late healing periods, contributing to tendon remodeling especially restoration of gliding surface. Proliferation of tenocytes is minimal in these stages. Apoptosis of cells is very prominent in adhesions and at the tendon-adhesion gliding interface. Edema in subcutaneous tissue and the tendon is an inevitable biologic process, contributing substantially to the resistance to tendon gliding. Major annular pulleys may greatly resist gliding of a repaired and swelling tendon. Experimentally, edema of the subcutaneous tissues contributed 20% to 25%, the intact A2 pulley 30%, extensor tendons 15%, and joint stiffness etc of 25% to 30% of total resistance to the gliding of the flexor tendon. Tendon bulkiness (swelling and surgical repairs) also greatly contributes to resistance. The contribution made by each of the earlier mentioned factors changes dynamically with time elapsed since surgery and the position of finger flexion. The overall resistance to tendon motion is progressively increased when the digit is markedly flexed. Careful consideration of the contributing factors and their dynamics provides insight into strategies to reduce repair rupture and maximize tendon gliding through surgery and postoperative motion protocols.

REFERENCES

1. Potenza AD. Tendon healing within the flexor digital sheath in the dog. J Bone Joint Surg Am 1962;44:49–64.
2. Potenza AD. Critical evaluation of flexor-tendon healing and adhesion formation within artificial digital sheaths. J Bone Joint Surg Am 1963;45:1217–33.
3. Jones ME, Mudera V, Brown RA, et al. The early surface cell response to flexor tendon injury. J Hand Surg Am 2003;28:221–30.
4. Ingraham JM, Weber RA, Childs EW. Intrinsic tendon healing requires the recycling of tendon collagen fibril segments. J Hand Surg Eur 2011;36:154–5.
5. Yuan J, Murrell GA, Wei AQ, et al. Apoptosis in rotator cuff tendonopathy. J Orthop Res 2002;20: 1372–9.
6. Nell EM, van der Merwe L, Cook J, et al. The apoptosis pathway and the genetic predisposition to Achilles tendinopathy. J Orthop Res 2012;30: 1719–24.
7. Lundgreen K, Lian OB, Engebretsen L, et al. Tenocyte apoptosis in the torn rotator cuff: a primary or secondary pathological event? Br J Sports Med 2011;45:1035–9.
8. Lui PP, Cheuk YC, Hung LK, et al. Increased apoptosis at the late stage of tendon healing. Wound Repair Regen 2007;15:702–7.
9. Wu YF, Chen CH, Cao Y, et al. Molecular events of cellular apoptosis and proliferation in the early tendon healing period. J Hand Surg Am 2010;35:2–10.
10. Wu YF, Zhou YL, Mao WF, et al. Cellular apoptosis and proliferation in the middle and late intrasynovial tendon healing periods. J Hand Surg Am 2012;37: 209–16.
11. Wong JK, Lui YH, Kapacee Z, et al. The cellular biology of flexor tendon adhesion formation: an old problem in a new paradigm. Am J Pathol 2009; 175:1938–51.
12. Chang J, Most D, Stelnicki E, et al. Gene expression of transforming growth factor beta-1 in rabbit zone II flexor tendon wound healing: evidence for dual mechanisms of repair. Plast Reconstr Surg 1997; 100:937–44.
13. Tsubone T, Moran SL, Amadio PC, et al. Expression of growth factors in canine flexor tendon after laceration in vivo. Ann Plast Surg 2004;53:393–7.
14. Chen CH, Cao Y, Wu YF, et al. Tendon healing in vivo: gene expression and production of multiple growth factors in early tendon healing period. J Hand Surg Am 2008;33:1834–42.
15. Chang J, Thunder R, Most D, et al. Studies in flexor tendon wound healing: neutralizing antibody to TGF-beta 1 increase postoperative range of motion. Plast Reconstr Surg 2000;105:148–55.
16. Schoof CR, Botelho EL, Izzotti A, et al. MicroRNAs in cancer treatment and prognosis. Am J Cancer Res 2012;2:414–33.
17. Chen CH, Zhou YL, Wu YF, et al. Effectiveness of microRNA in down-regulation of TGF-beta gene expression in digital flexor tendons of chickens: in vitro and in vivo study. J Hand Surg Am 2009; 34:1777–84.
18. Tang JB, Cao Y, Zhu B, et al. Adeno-associated virus-2-mediated bFGF gene transfer to digital flexor tendons significantly increases healing strength. an in vivo study. J Bone Joint Surg Am 2008;90: 1078–89.

19. Thomopoulos S, Kim HM, Das R, et al. The effects of exogenous basic fibroblast growth factor on intrasynovial flexor tendon healing in a canine model. J Bone Joint Surg Am 2010;92:2285–93.

20. Yao J, Korotkova T, Smith RL. Viability and proliferation of pluripotential cells delivered to tendon repair sites using bioactive sutures–an in vitro study. J Hand Surg Am 2011;36:252–8.

21. Bates SJ, Morrow E, Zhang AY, et al. Mannose-6-phosphate, an inhibitor of transforming growth factor-beta, improves range of motion after flexor tendon repair. J Bone Joint Surg Am 2006;88:2465–72.

22. Cao Y, Tang JB. Investigation of resistance of digital subcutaneous edema to gliding of the flexor tendon: an in vitro study. J Hand Surg Am 2005;30:1248–54.

23. Cao Y, Tang JB. Resistance to motion of flexor tendons and digital edema: an in vivo study in a chicken model. J Hand Surg Am 2006;31:1645–51.

24. Xie RG, Cao Y, Xu XF, et al. The gliding force and work of flexion in the early days after primary repair of lacerated flexor tendons: an experimental study. J Hand Surg Eur 2008;33:192–6.

25. Halikis MN, Manske PR, Kubota H, et al. Effect of immobilization, immediate mobilization, and delayed mobilizationon the resistance to digital flexion using a tendon injury model. J Hand Surg Am 1997;22:464–72.

26. Zhao C, Amadio PC, Paillard P, et al. Digital resistance and tendon strength during the first week after flexor digitorum profundus tendon repair in a canine model in vivo. J Bone Joint Surg Am 2004;86:320–7.

27. Zhao C, Amadio PC, Tanaka T, et al. Short-term assessment of optimal timing for postoperative rehabilitation after flexor digitorum profundus tendon repair in a canine model. J Hand Ther 2005;18:322–9.

28. Tang JB, Shi D, Zhang QG. Biomechanical and histologic evaluation of tendon sheath management. J Hand Surg Am 1996;21:900–8.

29. Tang JB. The double sheath system and tendon gliding in zone 2C. J Hand Surg Br 1995;20:281–5.

30. Buonocore S, Sawh-Martinez R, Emerson JW, et al. The effects of edema and self-adherent wrap on the work of flexion in a cadaveric hand. J Hand Surg Am 2012;37:1349–55.

31. Cao Y, Chen CH, Wu YF, et al. Digital oedema, adhesion formation and resistance to digital motion after primary flexor tendon repair. J Hand Surg Eur 2008;33:745–52.

32. Moriya T, Larson MC, Zhao C, et al. The effect of core suture flexor tendon repair techniques on gliding resistance during static cycle motion and load to failure: a human cadaver study. J Hand Surg Eur 2012;37:316–22.

33. Lee SK, Goldstein RY, Zingman A, et al. The effects of core suture purchase on the biomechanical characteristics of a multistrand locking flexor tendon repair: a cadaveric study. J Hand Surg Am 2010;35:1165–71.

34. Waitayawinyu T, Martineau PA, Luria S, et al. Comparative biomechanic study of flexor tendon repair using FiberWire. J Hand Surg Am 2008;33:701–8.

35. Lee SK. Modern tendon repair techniques. Hand Clin 2012;28:565–70.

36. Zhao C, Amadio PC, Zobitz ME, et al. Resection of the flexor digitorum superficialis reduces gliding resistance after zone II flexor digitorum profundus repair in vitro. J Hand Surg Am 2002;27:316–21.

37. Tang JB, Xu Y, Chen F. Impact of flexor digitorum superficialis on gliding function of the flexor digitorum profundus according to regions in zone II. J Hand Surg Am 2003;28:838–44.

38. Xu Y, Tang JB. Effects of superficialis tendon repairs on lacerated profundus tendons within or proximal to the A2 pulley: an in vivo study in chickens. J Hand Surg Am 2003;28:994–1001.

39. Kwai Ben I, Elliot D. "Venting" or partial lateral release of the A2 and A4 pulleys after repair of zone 2 flexor tendon injuries. J Hand Surg Br 1998;23:649–54.

40. Elliot D. Primary flexor tendon repair—operative repair, pulley management and rehabilitation. J Hand Surg Br 2002;27:507–13.

41. Tang JB. Clinical outcomes associated with flexor tendon repair. Hand Clin 2005;21:199–210.

42. Tang JB. Indications, methods, postoperative motion and outcome evaluation of primary flexor tendon repairs in Zone 2. J Hand Surg Eur 2007;32:118–29.

43. Tang JB. Tendon injuries across the world: treatment. Injury 2006;37:1036–42.

44. Tomaino M, Mitsionis G, Basitidas J, et al. The effect of partial excision of the A2 and A4 pulleys on the biomechanics of finger flexion. J Hand Surg Br 1998;23:50–2.

45. Mitsionis G, Bastidas JA, Grewal R, et al. Feasibility of partial A2 and A4 pulley excision: Effect on finger flexor tendon biomechanics. J Hand Surg Am 1999;24:310–4.

46. Tanaka T, Amadio PC, Zhao C, et al. The effect of partial A2 pulley excision on gliding resistance and pulley strength in vitro. J Hand Surg Am 2004;29:877–83.

47. Tang JB, Xie RG, Cao Y, et al. A2 pulley incision or one slip of the superficialis improves flexor tendon repairs. Clin Orthop Relat Res 2007;456:121–7.

48. Tang JB, Cao Y, Wu YF, et al. Effect of A2 pulley release on repaired tendon gliding resistance and rupture in a chicken model. J Hand Surg Am 2009;34:1080–7.

49. Cao Y, Tang JB. Strength of tendon repair decreases in the presence of an intact A2 pulley: biomechanical study in a chicken model. J Hand Surg Am 2009;34:1763–70.

50. Wu YF, Zhou YL, Tang JB. Relative contribution of tissue oedema and the presence of an A2 pulley to resistance to flexor tendon movement: an in vitro and in vivo study. J Hand Surg Eur 2012;37:310–5.

Current Practice of Primary Flexor Tendon Repair
A Global View

Jin Bo Tang, MD[a],*, Peter C. Amadio, MD[b],
Martin I. Boyer, MD[c], Robert Savage, MS, FRCS[d],
Chunfeng Zhao, MD[b], Michael Sandow, FRCS[e,f],
Steve K. Lee, MD[g], Scott W. Wolfe, MD[g]

KEYWORDS

- Flexor tendon • Primary repair • Strong surgical repair • Core sutures • Flexor pulley
- Pulley venting • Surgical techniques • Rehabilitation

KEY POINTS

- Primary or delayed flexor tendon repairs in the hand have become standard practice over the past 30 years; direct end-to-end repair in the digital sheath area using a multistrand core suture (4-strand, 6-strand, or 8-strand repair) has become widely adopted over the last 10 years.
- Although repair methods vary, basic principles include use of strong surgical repairs, slightly higher tension over the repair site, and ensuring sufficient core suture purchase (1.0 cm).
- 3-0 or 4-0 sutures are used for making core sutures, and 6-0 sutures are used for peripheral suturing. A strong core suture (6-strand or greater), made with proper tension over the repair site, may circumvent the use of peripheral sutures.
- In the past 10 years, the policy for preservation of the pulleys has been revolutionized. A part of the A2 pulley can be incised to free tendon motion, or the entire A4 pulley may be incised to allow repair and tendon movement if other pulleys are intact.
- Combined active-passive motion regimes are the mainstay of postoperative care, but the details of exercise protocols vary greatly. Rubber-band traction has been almost abandoned, and purely passive motion has declined in popularity.

Lacerated flexor tendons, especially those in the digital sheath area, were largely not considered candidates for primary surgical repair in the first half of the twentieth century. Primary repair of the flexor tendon in the digital sheath area was established in the 1970s to the 1980s, following conceptual changes brought about by pioneers such as Claude Verdan and Harold Kleinert in the 1960s. Although indications for primary repair are similar to those described decades ago, the surgical techniques, concepts regarding treatment of sheath and pulleys, and methods of postoperative care changed considerably. The ultimate goals remain to achieve close-to-ideal functional restoration and predictable clinical outcomes.

[a] Department of Hand Surgery, Affiliated Hospital of Nantong University, 20 West Temple Road, Nantong 226001, Jiangsu, China; [b] Department of Orthopedics, Mayo Clinic, Rochester, MN 55905, USA; [c] Department of Orthopedic Surgery, Washington University, St Louis, MO 63110, USA; [d] Trauma and Orthopedic Department, Royal Gwent Hospital, Cardiff Road, Newport NP20 2UB, Gwent, UK; [e] Department of Orthopedics and Trauma, Royal Adelaide Hospital, North Terrace, Adelaide SA 5000, Australia; [f] Physiotherapy Department, Royal Adelaide Hospital, Adelaide, Australia; [g] Hospital for Special Surgery, Weill Cornell Medical College, 535 East 70th Street, New York, NY 10021, USA
* Corresponding author.
E-mail address: jinbotang@yahoo.com

Hand Clin 29 (2013) 179–189
http://dx.doi.org/10.1016/j.hcl.2013.02.003
0749-0712/13/$ – see front matter © 2013 Elsevier Inc. All rights reserved.

hand.theclinics.com

This article reviews the evolution of treatment methods and provides global views and details of the surgical methods and rehabilitation regimes used in major hand units across the world. The surgical principles and key technical considerations underlying these diverse treatment options are also summarized.

CURRENT PRACTICE ACROSS THE GLOBE
United States and North America

Although exact statistical data are not available from members of the American Society for Surgery of the Hand (ASSH), in the last decade there has been a clear technical shift in core tendon repair, from conventional 2-strand core sutures to methods with 4 or more suture strands. The current methods of digital flexor tendon repair in the United States have been developed by units that have spent decades in the development of repair methods.

Mayo Clinic
The current practice is (1) use of a 3-0, low-friction suture material, with a 4-strand high-strength repair; (2) low-friction suture design, such as the modified Pennington, with locking loops[1]; (3) a running epitendinous finishing suture; (4) recourse to pulley trimming,[2,3] or excision of 1 slip of the flexor digitorum superficialis (FDS)[4] in cases of difficulty in tendon gliding in zone 2; (5) early motion after a few days' delay; (6) starting with a modified synergistic therapy,[5] and (8) progression to active motion as healing progresses.

The preference of Dr Amadio is a modified Pennington suture design for the core suture, because it locks the loops definitively by coming out of the tendon dorsally. He uses 2 such core sutures, made with either 3-0 or 4-0 TiCron, depending on tendon size. Other surgeons use double Tsuge sutures, made with 3-0 or 4-0 Supramid, with 1 on each side of the tendon, being sure to keep the surface loops lateral, to minimize friction. Some others prefer the modified Kessler repair.

The peripheral sutures used at Mayo commonly are simple running sutures of 6-0 nylon or Prolene, although Dr Amadio does prefer a running locking suture. The Lin locking suture is not used clinically, because it is difficult to perform and it causes more friction than other peripheral sutures.

There is no standard rehabilitation protocol used by all surgeons following tendon repair at the Mayo Clinic, and the specific details depend on the nature of the injury. They see many complex injuries in their practice, which receives referrals from a large agricultural region. Some of these patients return home for aftercare, and trained hand therapists may or may not be readily accessible. For a clean-cut injury in zone 2, the patient is initially placed in an extension block splint with the wrist and metacarpophalangeal (MCP) joints flexed. The Mayo Clinic no longer uses rubber-band (Kleinert) traction to the finger tips.

Passive motion is typically started using a modified synergistic protocol[5] combined with passive joint mobilization within 3 to 5 days after surgery,[6] and this progresses to place-and-hold exercises once the finger joints are supple. In this protocol, the patient comes out of the splint to actively flex the wrist and extend the fingers simultaneously. Then, while keeping the MCP joints extended, the interphalangeal (IP) joints are flexed (for the first few days passively, then later actively) and the wrist is actively extended. The patient comes out of the splint for exercises, usually several times each day. Usually by 3 weeks the patients have begun gentle active-motion exercises, including both fist and hook grip positions. The splint can usually be discarded by 6 weeks, and the patient can begin light resistive exercises, progressing to heavier use gradually over the next 6 weeks. Most patients are dismissed from care by week 10 or 12 if they are doing well. If not, other modalities such as ultrasound or stretching may be added.

Washington University (St Louis, MO)
The current practice in this unit is as follows: (1) use of a 3-0 or 4-0 low-friction suture material such as a looped braided caprolactam, with an 8-strand Gelberman-Winters core suture technique[7]; (2) placement of a single knot within the repair site; (3) a simple running epitendinous suture of 5-0 or 6-0 Prolene placed deeply across the tenorrhaphy site; (4) early motion using a synergistic protocol combining wrist flexion with active finger extension against a dorsal block, and finger flexion (passive, with a gentle active component) combined with active wrist extension.

At Washington University, surgeons prefer to use a Gelberman-Winters core suture technique, using the 3-0 or 4-0 braided caprolactam suture (Supramid) for the following 2 reasons: first, it allows for the passage of 2 suture strands with the single passage of the needle, and, second, the tapered design of the needle minimizes damage to the tendon during core suture insertion. If an 8-strand core suture is not possible because of small cross-sectional tendon area (such as at the A4 pulley or distal to it, or in the small finger), then a 4-strand modified Kessler pattern is used followed by an epitendinous suture. Based on the data of Diao and colleagues[8] and Nelson and colleagues,[9] they prefer to use a simple running epitendinous suture of 6-0 Prolene placed 2 mm from the tenorrhaphy site and also deeply within the tendon.

They routinely use a synergistic wrist protocol for patients who are able to participate actively in postoperative therapy. A hinged brace is used, which allows simultaneous synergistic motion of the digits and of the wrist. This protocol is based on experiments done in a clinically relevant in vivo canine model, which showed that this protocol provides a lower level of proximal musculotendinous force (and therefore less gap formation) and also an increased level of intrasynovial repair site excursion (so as to minimize repair site adhesions).[10] For patients unable to participate reliably in such a protocol or patients with isolated flexor pollicis longus tendon (FPL) lacerations, a modified Duran place-and-hold protocol is used.

Passive motion is typically started using a modified synergistic protocol combined with passive joint mobilization within 2 days following repair. The initial focus is on passive motion and edema control by means of digital wraps. The progression is similar to that described for the Mayo Clinic. The splint is discontinued once the repair site has accrued enough strength to withstand active-motion therapy (around 6 weeks). Resisted motion and strengthening do not begin until 10 to 12 weeks have elapsed from the time of repair.

Hospital for Special Surgery (New York)

Surgeons (Drs Lee SK and Wolfe SW) at Hospital for Special Surgery use a cross-locked cruciate as the core suture[11] with a braided nonabsorbable suture such as 3-0 or 4-0 FiberWire (Arthrex, Naples, FL) or 3-0 or 4-0 Ethibond. The suture span (middle of the X from the lacerated end of the tendon) is 10 mm (7 mm minimum) for optimal biomechanical performance.[12,13] This span is followed with a circumferential suture with either the interlocking horizontal mattress suture method with 6-0 Prolene or a running lock suture with a suture span of 2 mm (**Fig. 1**A, C).[14] The combination repair of cross-locked cruciate interlocking horizontal mattress (CLC-IHM) has an ultimate strength of 111 N, 2-mm gap force of 90 N, and only a 5% increase in work of flexion, the lowest increase in work of flexion reported to date.[12]

The CLC-IHM repair can be technically demanding, but the benefits of a strong repair with minimal bulk are worth the effort. The core suture should start in the center and dorsally; this ensures that the suture knot will not protrude out of the repair site and catch on pulleys. The tendon ends must be perfectly opposed before starting the suturing, which can be accomplished with 25-gauge needles placed in both tendon ends

approximately 15 to 20 mm from the cut ends of the tendon. Once the second cross lock is placed and tightened, the tendon ends hold their position, meaning that the ends cannot be overopposed, which would bulge the tendon ends otherwise. If the tendon ends are gapped at the beginning of the suture process, the tendon ends cannot be opposed when using a braided suture. Each cross lock should be cinched tightly like shoestrings as the surgeon proceeds. The core suture knot has 6 throws/hitches (surgeon's knot plus 4 half hitches). Use of a circumferential suture is imperative to prevent gapping. Dr Lee prefers the interlocking horizontal mattress suture; Dr Wolfe uses a running lock method.

With this repair method, patients can be moved early.[12,13] The strength of the repair in an early motion protocol increases from time zero; only when tendons are immobilized postoperatively do they get weaker temporarily before getting stronger (the softening effect). Based on the work of Cao and Tang,[15] we strive to have patients start motion at 4 to 5 days. Synergistic hand motion (wrist flexion with active digital extension, wrist extension with active fist), followed by tip-to-palm place and hold, hook fist positioning, and intrinsic plus exercises are key exercises. The patients commence these exercises at 4 to 5 days. Blocking exercises start at 4 weeks, strengthening at 8 weeks, unrestricted regular activity at 6 months, and contact sport at 9 months.

Stanford University Medical Center (Palo Alto)

Surgeons (Dr Chang and others) used the epitendinous suture-first method. A continuous epitendinous suture is added with 6-0 nylon, followed by a 4-strand core repair (modified Strickland), consisting of a locking Kessler repair and a 2-strand horizontal mattress suture using 3-0 or 4-0 sutures. The knot of the locking Kessler repair is buried under the tendon surface. The tendon purchase is 2 mm for epitendinous stitches and 1 cm for core stitches. Combined passive and active motion is prescribed for 6 weeks after surgery. The original Strickland repair (4 strands) shown in **Fig. 1** is used in some other units.

The increasingly popular wide-awake approach for flexor tendon surgery was developed by Lalonde in Canada. This approach allows intraoperative assessment of tendon gliding and gapping between the repaired ends. Dr Lalonde and colleagues typically use a 4-strand core suture and midrange active motion after surgery.

Australia

The current practice in tendon repair in Australia has been in parallel with international experience,

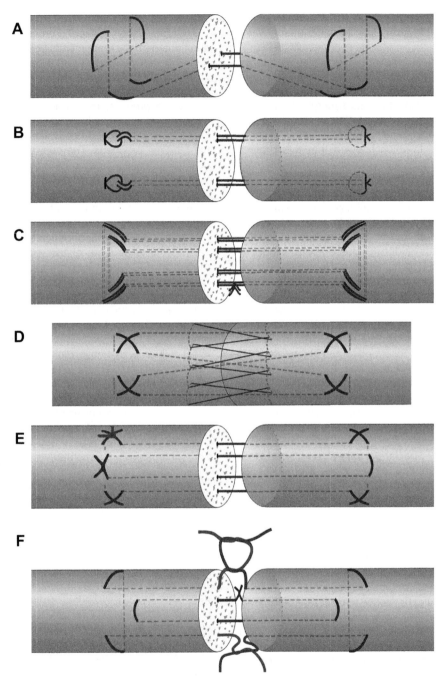

Fig. 1. Core suture methods used in different units: (*A*) modified Pennington suture (*lateral view*), (*B*) 4-strand double Tsuge suture. Both (*A*) and (*B*) are used in the Mayo Clinic. (*C*) Eight-strand Gelberman-Winters suture used in Washington University in St Louis (MO). (*D*) Cruciate repair used in the Hospital of Special Surgery, New York (NY). The interlocking peripheral suture is also shown. (*E*) A modified Strickland, a 4-strand repair made up of a locking Kessler repair and a horizontal mattress suture, used in the Stanford University Medical Center. (*F*) Strickland suture. (*B*–*F*) The repair in anterior view.

with important local contributions by Walsh, Tonkin, and Sandow, and their associated groups.[16–20] Although the modified Kessler has been the workhorse in the past, a recent survey in Australia identified that around 80% of hand surgeons in that country are now using a multi-strand (greater than 2 strands) core repair, most of which are the 4-strand single cross-grasp modification of the Savage technique (Adelaide repair).[19,20] The use of a multistrand surgical repair and a fully active-mobilization postrepair protocol has been a standard in several centers. The single cross-grasp 4-stand Adelaide repair was introduced into routine use in several centers in 1994,[20] and is now a dominant repair technique nationally. The technique of epitendinous repair varies from a simple loop to a stronger Silfverskiold repair, depending on surgeon preference and tendon dimensions.

With the introduction of stronger repairs allied with improved training, there has been a notable reduction in the number of cases needing secondary surgery in Australia. If secondary tendon grafting is required, there has been an increased use of active mobilization in conjunction with single-stage tendon grafting.

United Kingdom and Other European Countries

United Kingdom

A survey of British Society of Surgery of the Hand (BSSH) members was performed in 2011 to evaluate current practice for primary flexor tendon repair among its members. Sixty-one responded with a 2:1 split between orthopedic-trained and plastic-trained hand surgeons. The number of cases per respondent ranged from fewer than 5 cases per year (in 18 respondents), often the work of individual surgeons, to more than 30 cases per year (in 5 respondents), being either individual surgeons or, in a few instances, groups of surgeons.

Four-strand core sutures were most popular (46 respondents), a 2-strand repair was used by 15, 6-strand repair by 5, and 8-strand repair by 1 surgeon. There was a predominance of double Kessler, Adelaide, and Strickland users. The most popular core suture material was Prolene (31 respondents), followed by braided polyester (23), nylon (9), FiberWire (1), and Polydioxanone (PDS) (1). Twenty-nine used a simple peripheral suture, 17 the Silfverskiold suture, and 10 a locking peripheral suture.

Fifty-nine respondents performed partial A2 and A4 pulley venting, 2 never vented the pulleys, and 6 sometimes vented all of the A4 pulleys. Twenty never closed the sheath, 22 closed part of the sheath, and 6 always closed the whole sheath.

Forty-four surgeons used controlled active mobilization postoperatively, 2 used passive movement, and 4 used active mobilization. Mobilization was commenced within a few days to a week in all cases. Forty-two continued splintage for 6 weeks, with several 2 weeks shorter or

longer. The most popular wrist splint angle was 0° (29 respondents), with 16 favoring various flexion angles up to 40° and 7 various extension angles up to 30°. The preferred MCP splint angle was between 40° and 80° in most cases, with a few greater or less than this, and proximal interphalangeal splint angle was mainly near fully extended, with 2 flexed to 40°.

In considering repair principles, most surgeons thought sutures were necessary in restoring function but were concerned about the effect on tendon health. A few were strongly opposed to thick suture sizes, bulky knots, and multistrand repairs, but many accepted the need for multistrand repairs.

Among members of BSSH, there was wide acceptance of the practical benefits of early mobilization to reduce adhesion and improve range of motion, but there was concern about the risk of tendon rupture. All respondents considered the effects of tendon repair gapping/separation to be deleterious to tendon mobility and results, with concern about associated adhesion, snagging on pulleys, and incipient rupture.

In the United Kingdom, most surgeons embraced the current trend of creating repair robustness either with 4-strand or 6-strand core repair, or with Silfverskiold, locking, or simple peripheral sutures. Many found this to be an uncomfortable decision based on their training and on laboratory work on tendon healing, but most thought that the advantage of multistrand repair strength outweighed the theoretic risks of tendon damage from excessive suture material and tendon handling.

University of Bern, Switzerland

In Bern, a 6-strand Lim-Tsai repair (4-0 looped nylon) followed by a simple running peripheral suture (**Fig. 2**), is a common way to repair the flexor digitorum profundus (FDP) tendon.[21,22] Postoperative care consists of pure active, partial active–partial passive, or pure passive motion (with more robust protective immobilization with plaster or splint), depending on the severity of the injuries to the tendon and surrounding tissues, hand and forearm edema, and damage to other structures (such as fractures and soft tissue loss).[22]

Verona University, Italy

The accepted practice for repairing the FDP tendon is a 4-strand core suture with a single knot using a 3-0 or 4-0 nylon suture. This suture consists of 4 parallel strands tied with a single knot embedded between the two tendon ends. There are 4 grasping anchor points in each of the two tendon stumps (see **Fig. 2**). This 4-strand method was described

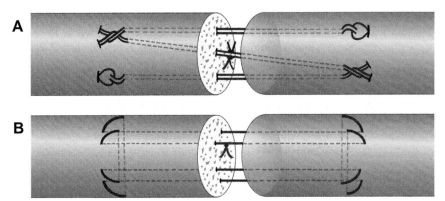

Fig. 2. Core suture methods used in (*A*) University of Bern, and (*B*) Verona University.

by Dubert in Pontault-Combault, France, and also used by Dr Adani in Verona, Italy. The core suture is strengthened by a simple running peripheral suture made with 5-0 or 6-0 nylon, which also prevents impingement of the repair site under the pulleys. In case of sharp lacerations in zone 2, they prefer to repair both FDP and FDS tendons. The FDS is repaired with a 2-strand modified Kessler or with a simple Tsuge loop suture. In cases of complex injuries (eg, replantation or mutilating injuries), only the FDP is repaired.

A protective back slab is replaced with a splint with the wrist in neutral position, the MCP joints flexed about 50°, and IP joints in extension. Five days after surgery, active-motion exercises are started. The splint is maintained for 5 weeks.

In Italy, the FDP tendon injury in zone 1 or distal zone 2 is often treated using the Mantero technique (a pull-out repair over the fingertip). This method has been popular in this country. Early active motion is important in achieving good results with this technique.

China and Other Asian Countries

Repair methods for the lacerated FDP tendon have been influenced by the technique of the Tusge looped suture,[23] though modified Kessler and its 4-strand variants are also popular. In Japan, looped-suture tendon repair dominates as the method of flexor tendon repair. This method of tendon repair (and its variants) is also popular in Singapore and China. However, in mainland China, more variations of tendon repair methods are seen. Hand surgeons use 2-strand, 4-strand, and 6-strand repair methods; repairs using looped sutures and conventional single-stranded suture are also common. Methods at 2 hand centers in the coastal areas of mainland China, and Chang Gung Memorial Hospital in Taiwan are presented later.

Chang Gung Memorial Hospital

In this hospital, 4-0 PDS sutures are regularly used for core sutures of the flexor tendon and 6-0 nylon is used for epitendinous running sutures. Though 4-strand core sutures are most common, 6 strands are used occasionally in the forearm. A part of the A2 pulley or the A4 pulley is vented on the lateral border if necessary to allow tendon gliding after repair. Passive motion is initiated in the first 2 weeks after surgery, followed by protective active motion from 2 to 4 weeks, and active motion after 4 weeks.

At Chang Gung Memorial Hospital, the same repair methods are used for primary tendon repair in replantation surgery as are used primary repair of a simple laceration.

Nantong University

The senior surgeons in this unit use a 6-strand repair with looped nylon sutures (**Fig. 3**)[24–26] for FDP or FPL tendon repair, or a 4-strand repair for FDS tendon repair. A part of the A2 pulley or the entire A4 pulley is vented through the volar midline to free gliding of the repaired tendon. The M-shaped 6-strand repair[25,26] replaced the original triple Tsuge repair[24] because the newer method reduces the number of sutures used and likely simplifies the surgery, although both the earlier method and the current one produced the same clinical outcomes. The FDS is usually not repaired if the site of damage is covered by the A2 pulley. Either 3-0 or 4-0 sutures are used for making the core suture, and 6-0 suture is used for the peripheral suture. Other 4-strand core repairs are also used in repairing the flat FDS tendon or the tendons in the palm and distal forearm.[27]

At Nantong University, patients are instructed to start active extension and midrange active (within or upto one-half to two-thirds range) flexion starting from day 4 or 5. Digital edema is common for

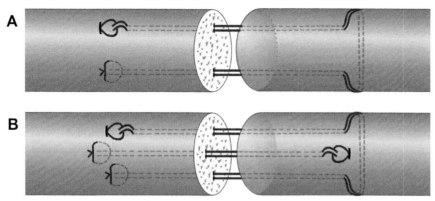

Fig. 3. Two methods, (*A*) the 4-strand suture and (*B*) the 6-strand repair (M-Tang), used in Nantong University.

the first few days and motion of the digits may induce pain and bleeding. Delaying motion for a few days logically would not increase adhesion formation (adhesions do not form in the first week after surgery) and do not increase the chance of joint stiffness, but it does reduce the workload of therapists and discomfort of the patient.[15,28] In the first 2.5 to 3 weeks, the emphasis is placed on full extension of the IP joints, but active digital flexion is necessary only over the initial one-third to two-thirds of finger flexion range (ie, partial active-motion or midrange active-motion regime).[26] After 2.5 to 3 weeks, the splint is changed to keep the wrist in a functional position, and range of active flexion is increased (gradually and not against external resistance or excessive internal resistance). A full range of active flexion is encouraged at weeks 4 and 5. The patient actively moves the hand without splint protection after week 6 and returns to normal use in weeks 8 to 10.[26]

In another unit, the Wuxi Hand Surgery Hospital, the U-shaped (4-strand) core repair is used for simple zone 2 repairs and in repairs associated with replantation (see **Fig. 3**).[29,30] The 4-strand repair is supplemented with a variety of robust peripheral sutures (made with 5-0 or 6-0 suture). Combined early active motion without place and hold is the standard method of postoperative care in this unit.

Because of the geographic proximity of Vladivostok in Russia to China, the Korean peninsula, and Japan, the method used at Vladivostok Medical University has an Asian influence. Looped suture lines are commonly used for tendon repair in this unit. Early combined passive-active motion starts a few days after surgery. Research into modification of tendon repair methods is pursued by senior surgeon Dr Alexander Zolotov.[31]

Table 1 summarizes the current practice in some of the leading hand units. Details of surgical methods and postoperative care about 2 of the units on the list are available separately.[32,33] No repair ruptures have been reported with the wide-awake surgical approach by Lalonde and colleagues[33] or with a 6-strand core suture–only repair by Elliot and Giesen.[32]

SUMMARY OF CHANGES AND CURRENT PRACTICE

A striking finding in the global review of practice is the variations in methods used in individual units and by different surgeons. Nevertheless, the commonalities are clear and straightforward. The review suggests that treatment guidelines, rather than details of techniques, are essentially identical in current practice. Surgeons and therapists adopt methods that they are comfortable with and find reasonable, but there are common underlying principles:

1. Primary or delayed repairs continue to be a standard practice in digital flexor tendon repair. Direct end-to-end repair using multi-strand core suture (4-strand, 6-strand, or 8-strand repair) has been increasingly used in the last 10 years.

2. Although current repair methods vary, some principles are universal, such as using strong core sutures, ensuring knot security, using secure suture-tendon junctions, creating tighter tension over the repair site,[34] and ensuring sufficient core suture purchase (1.0 cm).[35,36]

3. 3-0 or 4-0 sutures are used for making core sutures, and 6-0 sutures are used for peripheral sutures.[36] The importance of adding peripheral sutures to prevent gapping of the repair site is stressed by many surgeons and is supported by in vivo and ex vivo biomechanical studies.[8,9,13,14] In contrast,

Table 1
The methods used currently in some hand surgery units in direct end-to-end flexor tendon repairs

Units	Core Sutures	Peripheral Sutures	Postoperative Motion	Country
Mayo Clinic	Modified Pennington, double Tsuge, double Kessler	Simple running or simple locking	Synergistic hand motion Place and hold, active motion, week 3 onward	United States
Washington University, St Louis (MO)	8-strand looped suture repair (ie, Gelberman-Winters)	Simple running	Synergistic hand motion Passive motion Active motion, week 3 onward	United States
Hospital for Special Surgery, New York (NY)	Cruciate	Interlocking or running locking	Place and hold Wrist tenodesis with active extension/flexion	United States
Stanford University, Palo Alto (CA)	Modified Kessler plus 2-strand horizontal mattress suture	Simple running	Place and hold Active motion, week 4 onward	United States
Saint John Regional Hospital	Double Kessler	Simple running	Midrange active protocol Abandon place and hold	Canada
University of Bern	6-strand Lim/Tsai	Simple running	Green/yellow/red protocols chosen by severity of injuries/quality of surgery[22]	Switzerland
Verona University	4-strand Kessler	Simple running	Active-motion protocol	Italy
Broomfield Hospital, Chelmsford	4-strand Evans/Smith 6-strand Tang	Simple running None	Midrange active protocol	United Kingdom
Chang Gung Memorial Hospital	4-strand, mostly 6-strand, occasionally	Simple running	Passive motion, 2 wk Active motion, week 3 onward	China
Nantong University	6-strand M-Tang, 4-strand U-shaped, cruciate	Interrupted or simple running	Midrange active protocol	China

a recent case series shows that a strong core suture (6 strands or greater), made with appropriate tension over the repair site, may avoid the need for peripheral sutures.[32]

4. Recent laboratory findings have been translated into clinical practice, including trimming of the partially lacerated tendon ends to reduce tendon gliding resistance, excision of 1 slip of the FDS, starting the postoperative motion a few days after surgery (rather than the next day),[15,34] ensuring that tendon movement relies on smooth tendon gliding rather than greater force during rehabilitation, and avoiding extreme active flexion during early active tendon motion.[26]

5. In the past 10 years, theories about treatment of the pulleys have changed.[26,37] A part of the A2 pulley can be incised to free tendon motion, and the entire A4 pulley may be incised to allow repair and tendon movement if other pulleys and the major part of the sheath are intact. Complete closure of the sheath is not considered necessary by most surgeons.

6. Combined active-motion/passive-motion regimes are the mainstay of postoperative care, but details of exercise protocols vary. Midrange active motion has emerged and has begun to be incorporated into active-motion regimes.

7. Synergistic wrist flexion and extension while the repaired finger is actively moved is now often incorporated to a motion regime. Rubber-band traction has mostly been abandoned.

8. Tendon repair methods in more severe hand trauma, such as replantation, are mostly the same as those used for a simple tendon laceration, but the FDS is not usually repaired.

9. New repair devices such as Teno Fix,[38] and suture materials like barbed sutures,[39] have not been adopted widely and are not currently used in the units reviewed in this article.

10. Distal tendon junctions can be achieved without a pull-out suture. The pull-out suture is no longer used and has been replaced by new methods in some units.

TECHNIQUES KEY TO SUCCESS

The aim of flexor tendon repair is near-complete restoration of range of active digital flexion, while avoiding rupture of the repair and formation of serious adhesions or joint contracture. Surgeons also aim to achieve predictable results. Following key guidelines is important in reaching these goals:

1. The surgical repair needs to be strong enough. Though there are a variety of methods to make a strong surgical repair, and it does not seem to matter which one surgeons choose. Strength can be achieved through a multistrand repair, large-caliber suture, or special devices that hold tendon ends tightly and strongly. The strength of the repair is essential, because the biological tendon healing strength does not increase for 2 to 3 weeks after surgery, and the risk of rupture is greatest during the first 2 weeks, when only the baseline surgical repair strength is holding the tendon ends together.

2. Avoiding gapping. Intraoperative validation of a tight, gap-free repair is important.[33] A certain tension across the repair site is helpful to resist gapping.[28] This tension can be achieved by using an efficient peripheral suture, a tighter core suture, or both.

3. Intraoperative testing of the repair site. Intraoperative testing of the repair site for possible gapping is important after completion of the repair.[26,33] This testing can be achieved by passively extending the finger,[26] or asking the patient to move actively during wide-awake surgery.[33]

4. Proper treatment of the major pulleys allows free gliding of the tendon. Major annular pulleys are the narrow parts along the tendon gliding path.[26] Venting of the narrow portions frees tendon gliding and avoids catching the repair site against the pulleys; however, overventing causes tendon bowstringing. Preservation of the entire A2 pulley can be harmful in some situations, such as when there are edematous tendon ends. Venting a part of the pulleys should only be done when other annular pulleys are intact. Surgeons should understand the intricate balance among the vented and preserved portions of the annular pulleys, and, of particular note, the entire A2 pulley should not be vented.

5. Active tendon movement with lower tension over the repair site. Both synergistic wrist motion and midrange active motion aim to reduce tension at the repair sites during active digital motion. Tension placed on tendons during active motion varies greatly with hand position and finger flexion ranges. Avoiding possible disruption of the repair by high-tensile load is a key to successful rehabilitation. Regimes can be designed to incorporate synergistic hand motion and midrange-only motion to reduce the tension, increasing the safety of tendon motion therapy.

It is now commonly understood that the following should be avoided: a weak repair, a loose repair (no tension across repair site), a repair with a short core suture purchase, repair gapping during intraoperative test with active tendon motion, constriction of the repair site under a tight A2 or A4 pulley, massive sutures that make the tendon surface rough, and a tendon that is bulky and is difficult to move after repair. Although any of these signals a poor repair, 2 or 3 such problems indicates that the repair is bound to disrupt or become stuck in serious adhesions, and heralds failure of the surgery.

ACKNOWLEDGMENTS

This article is an extensive and intimate international collaborative effort to summarize the current practice of digital flexor tendon repair across the world. The practice detail was provided by Drs Peter C. Amadio and Chunfeng Zhao for the Mayo Clinic, Dr Martin Boyer for Washington University (St Louis), Drs Steve K. Lee and Scott

Wolfe for Hospital for Special Surgery (New York), Dr James Chang for Stanford University (Palo Alto), Dr Michael Sandow for Australia, Mr Robert Savage for the United Kingdom, and Dr Jin Bo Tang for China and other Asian countries, Dr Chi Hung Lin (Taiwan), Dr Ester Veogelin (Bern, Switzerland), Dr Robert Adani (Verona, Italy), Dr Alexander Zolotov (Vladivostok, Russia). We thank members of the Australian Hand Surgery Society (AHSS) and BSSH for the survey information. This project was led and the article was finalized by Dr Jin Bo Tang.

REFERENCES

1. Momose T, Amadio PC, Zhao C, et al. Suture techniques with high breaking strength and low gliding resistance: experiments in the dog flexor digitorum profundus tendon. Acta Orthop Scand 2001;72: 635–41.

2. Moriya T, Thoreson AR, Zhao C, et al. The effects of oblique or transverse partial excision of the A2 pulley on gliding resistance during cyclic motion following zone II flexor digitorum profundus repair in a cadaveric model. J Hand Surg Am 2012;37: 1634–8.

3. Kutsumi K, Amadio PC, Zhao C, et al. Gliding resistance of the flexor pollicis longus tendon after repair: does partial excision of the oblique pulley affect gliding resistance? Plast Reconstr Surg 2006;118: 1423–8.

4. Zhao C, Amadio P, Zobitz M, et al. Resection of the flexor digitorum superficialis reduces gliding resistance after zone II flexor digitorum profundus repair in vitro. J Hand Surg Am 2002;27:316–21.

5. Zhao C, Amadio PC, Zobitz ME, et al. Effect of synergistic motion on flexor digitorum profundus tendon excursion. Clin Orthop Relat Res 2002;396:223–30.

6. Zhao C, Amadio PC, Paillard P, et al. Digital resistance and tendon strength during the first week after flexor digitorum profundus tendon repair in a canine model in vivo. J Bone Joint Surg Am 2004;86:320–7.

7. Winters SC, Gelberman RH, Woo SL, et al. The effects of multiple-strand suture methods on the strength and excursion of repaired intrasynovial flexor tendons: a biomechanical study in dogs. J Hand Surg Am 1998;23:97–104.

8. Diao E, Hariharan JS, Soejima O, et al. Effect of peripheral suture depth on strength of tendon repairs. J Hand Surg Am 1996;21:234–9.

9. Nelson GN, Potter R, Ntouvali E, et al. Intrasynovial flexor tendon repair: a biomechanical study of variations in suture application in human cadavera. J Orthop Res 2012;30:1652–9.

10. Boyer MI, Gelberman RH, Burns ME, et al. Intrasynovial flexor tendon repair. An experimental study comparing low and high levels of in vivo force during rehabilitation in canines. J Bone Joint Surg Am 2001; 83:891–9.

11. Barrie KA, Wolfe SW, Shean C, et al. A biomechanical comparison of multistrand flexor tendon repairs using an in situ testing model. J Hand Surg Am 2000;25:499–506.

12. Lee SK, Goldstein RY, Zingman A, et al. The effects of core suture purchase on the biomechanical characteristics of a multistrand locking flexor tendon repair: a cadaveric study. J Hand Surg Am 2010; 35:1165–71.

13. Lee SK. Modern tendon repair techniques. Hand Clin 2012;28:565–70.

14. Merrell GA, Wolfe SW, Kacena WJ, et al. The effect of increased peripheral suture purchase on the strength of flexor tendon repairs. J Hand Surg Am 2003;28:464–8.

15. Cao Y, Tang JB. Resistance to motion of flexor tendons and digital edema: an in vivo study in a chicken model. J Hand Surg Am 2006;31:1645–51.

16. Haddad R, Peltz TS, Walsh WR. Biomechanical evaluation of flexor tendon repair using barbed suture material: a comparative ex vivo study. J Hand Surg Am 2011;36(9):1565–6.

17. Peltz TS, Haddad R, Scougall PJ, et al. Influence of locking stitch size in a four-strand cross-locked cruciate flexor tendon repair. J Hand Surg Am 2011;36:450–5.

18. Strick MJ, Filan SL, Hile M, et al. Adhesion formation after flexor tendon repair: a histologic and biomechanical comparison of 2- and 4-strand repairs in a chicken model. J Hand Surg Am 2004;29:15–21.

19. Sandow MJ, McMahon M. Active mobilisation following single cross grasp four-strand flexor tenorrhaphy (Adelaide repair). J Hand Surg Eur 2011;36: 467–75.

20. Sandow MJ, McMahon M. Single-cross grasp six-strand repair for acute flexor tendon tenorrhaphy. Atlas Hand Clin 1996;1:41–64.

21. Hoffmann GL, Büchler U, Vögelin E. Clinical results of flexor tendon repair in zone II using a six-strand double-loop technique compared with a two-strand technique. J Hand Surg Eur 2008;33:418–23.

22. Vogelin E, Traber-Hoffmann G, van der Zypen V. Clinical primary flexor tendon repair and rehabilitation: the Bern experience. Treatment of rupture of primary flexor tendon repairs. In: Tang JB, Amadio PC, Guimberteau JC, et al, editors. Tendon surgery of the hand. Philadelphia: Elsevier Saunders; 2012. p. 116–24.

23. Tsuge K, Ikuta Y, Matsuishi Y. Repair of flexor tendons by intratendinous tendon suture. J Hand Surg Am 1977;2:436–40.

24. Tang JB, Shi D, Gu YQ, et al. Double and multiple looped suture tendon repair. J Hand Surg Br 1994; 19:699–703.

25. Tang JB. Clinical outcomes associated with flexor tendon repair. Hand Clin 2005;21:199–210.

26. Tang JB. Indications, methods, postoperative motion and outcome evaluation of primary flexor tendon repairs in Zone 2. J Hand Surg Eur 2007; 32:118–29.

27. Wu YF, Cao Y, Zhou YL, et al. Biomechanical comparisons of four-strand tendon repairs with double-stranded sutures: effects of different locks and suture geometry. J Hand Surg Eur 2011;36: 34–9.

28. Cao Y, Chen CH, Wu YF, et al. Digital oedema, adhesion formation and resistance to digital motion after primary flexor tendon repair. J Hand Surg Eur 2008;33:745–52.

29. Cao Y, Tang JB. Biomechanical evaluation of a four-strand modification of the Tang method of tendon repair. J Hand Surg Br 2005;30:374–8.

30. Ke ZS, Ri YJ, Shou KS, et al. A new 4-strand repair for flexor tendon repair: comparative biomechanical study. Chin J Hand Surg 2011;27:297–9 [in Chinese].

31. Zolotov AS. Primary repair of digital flexor tendons in several anatomic zones study. Questions of Reconstruct Plastic Surg 2012;15:19–25 [in Russia].

32. Elliot D, Giesen T. Primary flexor tendon surgery: the search for a perfect result. Hand Clin 2013;29: 191–206.

33. Lalonde DH, Martin A. Wide-awake flexor tendon repair and early tendon mobilization in zones 1 and 2. Hand Clin 2013;29:207–13.

34. Wu YF, Tang JB. Effects of tension across the tendon repair site on tendon gap and ultimate strength. J Hand Surg Am 2012;37:906–12.

35. Tang JB, Zhang Y, Cao Y, et al. Core suture purchase affects strength of tendon repairs. J Hand Surg Am 2005;30:1262–6.

36. Tang JB. Flexor tendon repair. In: Neligan P, Chang J, editors. Plastic surgery. Volume 6. Philadelphia: Elsevier Saunders; 2012. p. 178–205.

37. Elliot D. Primary flexor tendon repair-operative repair, pulley management and rehabilitation. J Hand Surg Br 2002;27:507–14.

38. Su BW, Solomons M, Barrow A, et al. Device for zone-II flexor tendon repair. A multicenter, randomized, blinded, clinical trial. J Bone Joint Surg Am 2005;87:923–35.

39. Zeplin PH, Zahn RK, Meffert RH, et al. Biomechanical evaluation of flexor tendon repair using barbed suture material: a comparative ex vivo study. J Hand Surg Am 2011;36:446–9.

Primary Flexor Tendon Surgery:
The Search for a Perfect Result

David Elliot, MA, FRCS*, Thomas Giesen, MD

KEYWORDS

- Flexor tendons • Zones • Subzones • Primary repair • Core and circumferential suture
- Venting pulleys • Rehabilitation • Rupture and adhesions

KEY POINTS

- The basis of modern management.
- An overview of the authors' unit's activity and research.
- Basic considerations of surgical repairs.
- Basic considerations of rehabilitation.
- The authors' current surgical practice, particularly in complicated situations.
- Management under difficult clinical conditions.

If a suture is not sufficiently strong to endure very early use, this connective tissue may seriously fix the tendon to the surrounding tissue … No splint is used. Active motion is started as soon as the patient has recovered from the anaesthetic.

—Harmer, Boston, 1917[1]

Repair of the divided flexor tendon to achieve normal, or near normal, function is an unsolved problem, with each result still uncertain. Over and above the actual technical difficulties of repairing the tendons, for a century this field has been dominated by the complications of adherence of repairs and rupture during early healing. Adhesion of the repairs occurs because the body creates a soup of fibrin-loaded edema in any area of healing, which Watson-Jones called "physiologic glue." The fibrin later converts to fibrous tissue to heal the injured tissues and achieve repair strength. This "gluing" process affects every structure in the vicinity, with little consideration of the particular need of certain tissues to glide within the interstitial connective tissue layers. Commonly, fibrin carried onto the dorsum of the digits with the edema fluid restricts movement of the digits into flexion after flexor tendon surgery both passively and actively, by tethering the extensor tendons to prevent their distal movement as the digits flex.[2] Adhesion can also occur anywhere along the flexor tendons with loss of active flexion and is a particular problem in the fingers, where the flexors are confined within the tendon sheath in a system as finely bored as the pistons in an engine. Avoiding this requires that the tendons be mobilized throughout the period immediately after repair, risking rupture, as the tendon repair takes about 3 months to achieve full strength.

THE BASIS OF MODERN SURGICAL TREATMENT

Although there is ongoing debate about the details of technique, the central tenet of modern flexor tendon surgery is to increase tendon healing, and to avoid adhesion formation between the repaired tendon and the surrounding tissues by making a repair that is strong enough to move within a few days of injury, as first suggested nearly 100 years ago and pioneered in the modern era by Verdan,

Conflict of Interest: None.
This research received no specific grant from any funding agency in the public, commercial, or not-for-profit sectors.
Hand Surgery Department, St Andrew's Centre for Plastic Surgery, Broomfield Hospital, Chelmsford, Essex, UK
* Corresponding author. Woodlands, Woodham Walter, Essex CM9 6LN, UK.
E-mail address: info@david-elliot.co.uk

Hand Clin 29 (2013) 191–206
http://dx.doi.org/10.1016/j.hcl.2013.03.001
0749-0712/13/$ – see front matter © 2013 Elsevier Inc. All rights reserved.

Young, and Harman and Kleinert.[1,3,4] There follows an unproven assumption that the results will be better with increasing early movement through the first 5 weeks, albeit within the protective environment of a dorsal splint, provided the sutures hold and rupture does not occur. Better tendon healing and adhesion limitation are 2 major goals of tendon surgery. Most methods to limit adhesions remain experimental.[5,6] In the authors' unit, the main interest over the last 20 years has been to eliminate the seemingly unconquerable rupture rate while maintaining a policy of enthusiastic early active mobilization.

FLEXOR TENDON REPAIR: AN OVERVIEW

In their unit, over the past 2 decades the authors have carried out approximately 90 to 100 simple primary flexor tendon repairs in all digits in adults each year, and have analyzed the outcomes and published several reports throughout this time.[7–17] The techniques of surgical repair and postoperative rehabilitation have been repeatedly modified, based on ongoing analysis of the clinical outcomes included in these reports. This article summarizes the authors' opinion of the basic essentials of surgical repairs and rehabilitation, followed by a brief description of their current surgical practice and preferred method of rehabilitation.

BASIC CONSIDERATIONS OF SURGICAL REPAIRS
Strengthening of Sutures: The Core Suture

The main drive of the mechanical way forward in the last 20 years has been by modification of the suturing of the divided tendon, in particular the core suturing (**Tables 1** and **2**). A variety of materials have been used but no best suture material identified. Various core-suture techniques have also been described over the years. Through the 1990s and the early years of this century, the Tajima and Strickland variations of the (2-strand) Kessler suture, whereby the knot, or knots, are buried in the tendon, were probably the most commonly used core-suture technique in Europe, whereas the Tsuge suture or, more recently, Tang's triple variation of it, were more likely to be used in the Far East.[18] Availability and historical factors, rather than measured strength, were probably the main determinants of which suture material and configurations were used in individual units and countries. As most of the published series of 2-strand core-suture zone 2 repairs in civilian populations from all over the world had roughly the same results, it would seem that most materials and most core-suture techniques in common use at that time worked equally well. Almost all had a rupture rate of between 2% and 9%, with an average of 5%. At the time, it was estimated that repairs needed to have a strength of 15 to 20 N to withstand early mobilization. However, in 1992 Schuind and colleagues measured forces of 120 N being transmitted through the flexor tendons at the wrist during strong pinch. In 1989, Savage and Risitano[19] increased the core-suture strength substantially using a Kessler-type suture with 6 strands across the tendon ends. This approach stimulated a great deal of laboratory work and publication of a smaller number of clinical articles, which has continued unremittingly since that time, leaving us with a very confusing multitude of core-suture options and no clear "winner." Savage's suture has seldom been surpassed for strength, but is difficult to insert. For this reason it is widely avoided in clinical practice. Research since might be viewed with a cynical eye as attempting to devise a multistrand core-suture technique with the strength advantage of the Savage suture while being more practical for clinical use. The array of options is well documented in a recent book chapter by Tang and colleagues.[20]

Although suture material does not seem to be of particular importance, Tang's review identifies 10 other factors of importance.[20] Modification of the number of strands of the core suture, and the various ways of achieving this, has attracted most attention, whereas another option, namely use of a larger caliber of core suture, is discussed rarely, although appearing simpler, at least at first glance. The benefits of increased suture size have been shown fairly convincingly in the laboratory.[21,22] However, thicker sutures become cumbersome to tie and the knot is bulky within the tendon with sutures thicker than 3/0 in size. This situation is avoided if the knot is taken out of the tendon and onto the tip of the digit, as in the Mantero technique,[23,24] probably based on a technique of distal tendon suture fixation described by Georgio Brunelli 20 years earlier. This technique originally used a 2/0 2-strand core suture with the suture attached through the proximal tendon using half of a Kirchmayer/Kessler suture[3,25] and to the distal tendon over a button at the tip of the digit, avoiding a knot within the flexor tendon itself. The technique and this suture size are still used routinely in many units in southern Europe, including Mantero's own unit, although some now use a smaller suture. Although the authors have no personal experience of the Mantero technique, it would seem most suited for use in cases where the flexor tendons are cut in the fingers beyond the A2 pulley, that is, in zone 1[12] and in Tang's zones 2A and 2B,[26] and in flexor pollicis longus (FPL)

Table 1
Methods and results of primary repair of simple finger flexor tendon injuries in adults from the authors' unit (*) and some other major reports

Authors,[Ref.] Year	Core Suture/Circumferential Suture/Rehabilitation	No. of Fingers	Zones	Excellent and Good Results (%)	Mechanical Rupture Rate (%)
Lister et al,[33] 1977	2-Strand/simple/KM	28 tendons	2	75	5
Small et al,[51] 1989	2-Strand/simple/EAM	117	2	77	9
Savage and Risitano,[19] 1989	6-Strand/simple/EAM	31	2	69	4
Saldana et al, 1991	2-Strand/simple/KM	60	2	93	5
Tang and Shi,[26] 1992	2-, 4-, 6-Strand/simple/EAM	54	2	81	5
Bainbridge et al,[59] 1994	i. 2-Strand/simple/KM ii. 2-Strand/simple/EAM	58 49	2 2	52 94	3 8
*Elliot et al,[7] 1994	2-Strand/simple/EAM	166	2	79	5
Tang et al,[18] 1994	4- or 6-Strand (Tsuge)/simple/EAM	51	1, 2	77 (White)	4
Silfverskiöld and May,[30] 1994	2-Strand/complex/KM + EAM + HOLD	55	2	96	4
Baktir et al,[61] 1996	i. 2-Strand/simple/KM ii. 2-Strand/simple/EAM	41 47	2 2	78 85	
Peck et al,[62] 1996	2-Strand/simple/EAM	82	2	71	12
*Harris et al,[10] 1999	2-strand/simple/EAM	397	2	—	4
Olivier,[63] 2001	i. 2-Strand/simple/KM ii. Towfigh device/simple/EAM with no splint	7 16	2 2	100 94	0 0
Baer et al,[32] 2003	2-Strand (Mantero)/simple/EAM	65	1, 2	91 (with FPL)	0
Klein,[64] 2003	4-strand/simple/KM	40	2	95	2
Golash et al,[65] 2003	i. 2-Strand/simple/EAM ii. 2-Strand/simple/EAM, ADCON	20 30	2 2	68 65	20 33
Peck et al,[66] 2004	2-Strand/simple/EAM	81	2	—	17
Su et al,[67] 2005	i. 4-Strand/simple/KM ii. Tenofix device/simple/KM	51 34	2 2	70 66	18 0
Hung et al,[68] 2005	2-Strand/simple/EAM	24	2	71	8
Caulfield et al,[69] 2008	i. Absorbable 4-strand/simple/EAM ii. Nonabsorbable 4-strand/EAM	72 129	1, 2 1, 2	74 74	8 2
Hoffmann et al,[70] 2008	6-Strand/simple/complex	51	2	78	2
Al-Qattan and Al-Turaiki,[71] 2009	6-Strand/simple/EAM	50	2	98	2
De Aguiar et al,[72] 2009	2-Strand/simple/EAM, Botulinum	34	2	87	0
Kitis et al,[73] 2009	i. 2-Strand/simple/KM ii. 2-Strand/simple/PM + HOLD	137 126	2 2	87 Excellent 75 Excellent	0 1
Trumble et al,[74] 2010	i. 4-Strand/simple/KM + PM ii. 4-Strand/simple/PM + HOLD	52 54	2	—	4 4
Georgescu et al,[75] 2011	2-Strand (Mantero)/simple/EAM	58	2	70	0
Sandow and McMahon,[76] 2011	4-Strand/simple/EAM	73	1, 2	71	5

Results were assessed by the original Strickland method[39] or the Buck-Gramcko method, except if given otherwise.

Abbreviations: EAM, Belfast or other early active mobilization (EAM) without rubber bands; FPL, flexor pollicis longus; IM, immobilized; KM, Kleinert-type mobilization with rubber bands; PM, Duran and Houser passive mobilization alone.

Table 2
Results of primary repair of simple flexor pollicis longus tendon injuries in the authors' unit (*) and some other units

Authors,[Ref.] Year	Core Suture/Circumferential Suture/Rehabilitation	No. of Thumbs	Zones	Excellent and Good Results (%)	Mechanical Rupture Rate (%)
*Sirotakova and Elliot,[11] 1999	i. 2-Strand/simple/EAM	30	1, 2	70 White, 73 Buck-G	17
	ii. 2-Strand/simple/EAM	39	1, 2	67 White, 72 Buck-G	15
	iii. 2-Strand/complex/EAM	49	1, 2	76 White, 80 Buck-G	8
Kasashima et al,[31] 2002	i. 2-Strand/simple/IM	16	1, 2, 3	50 (JSSH 1994)[a]	0
	ii. 2-Strand/simple/KM	13	1, 2, 3	77 (JSSH 1994)[a]	0
Peck et al,[66] 2004	2-Strand/simple/KM	23	1, 2	—	4
Baer et al,[32] 2003	2-Strand (Mantero)/simple/EAM	22	1, 2	91 Buck-G (with FDP)	0
*Sirotakova and Elliot,[15] 2004	4-Strand/complex/EAM	48	1, 2	73 White, 77 Buck-G	0
*Giesen et al,[17] 2007	6-Strand (Tang)/nil/EAM	49	1, 2	78 White, 82 Buck-G	0
Schaller,[77] 2010	2-Strand (Mantero)/simple/EAM	21	1, 2	66 Buck-G	0

Abbreviations: Buck-G, Buck-Gramcko method; EAM, Belfast or other early active mobilization (EAM); FDP, flexor digito-rum profundus; IM, immobilized; KM, Kleinert-type mobilization; PM, Duran and Houser passive mobilization alone.

[a] JSSH, criteria of Japanese Society for Surgery of the Hand (similar to the White assessment, uses interphalangeal range of motion only).

tendon division within the thumb, as the needles have to be passed within the distal tendon from the site of division to the top of the digit. This approach probably becomes more difficult as the length of distal tendon increases.

The FPL tendon was researched very little in the second half of the last century, but the extensive literature of an earlier era (1937–1960) clearly identified a much higher rupture rate after primary repair of the FPL than that after repairing the finger flexors.[27,28] Surgeons at that time recognized this and debated whether to repair this tendon by insertion of a tendon graft or by lengthening of the proximal tendon.[28] When the authors reported the results of zones 1 and 2 finger flexors in 1994[7] they also looked at the FPL results, and found an alarming rupture rate of 17% in 30 thumbs when mobilized in the Belfast regimen of active flexion/active extension of the repairs (**Table 2**). At that time, we recommended that this technique of mobilization should not be used in its present form after repair of the long thumb flexor. However, the authors realized that the higher rupture rate might make the FPL a good clinical model to test new sutures and suture techniques. Using this model, they were able to examine some of the new suture configurations being described at the time, in a series of clinical studies.[7,11,15,17] Although these articles elaborate an increasingly safer technique for dealing with division of the FPL tendon, they were undertaken largely to examine possible ways forward in respect of the finger flexors. Ultimately, these clinical experiments with the divided FPL achieved zero rupture rates using 2 different suture techniques, namely, a combination of a 4-strand core suture,[29] a Silf-verskiöld circumferential suture,[30] and Tang's triple-Tsuge suture repair.[18] This work showed that both the core and the circumferential suture could have a place in eliminating rupture. However, during the same period, 2 other units reported no mechanical ruptures of FPL repairs using 2-strand core sutures and simple circumferential repairs[31] or a Mantero repair,[32] albeit in small numbers of patients.

As seen in **Tables 1** and **2**, increasing the number of core-suture strands suggests a slight advantage in terms of reduction of ruptures of primary repairs, but not a total solution to the problem. However, nearly 50% of the articles published since 2000 report 50, or fewer than 50, repaired fingers. With such small numbers of cases, a difference of one rupture, more or less, would change the percentage ruptures by 2% or even 3%.

Strengthening of Sutures: The Circumferential Suture

The circumferential suture, which is never strictly "epitendinous," even in its simplest form, was originally introduced as an attempt to smooth down loose ends and improve gliding of the repair.[33] In 1986, Wade and colleagues[34] realized that it had considerable strength in itself. This notion led to a description of about 5 or 6 variants of the circumferential suture in the 1990s and several laboratory trials of the various alternatives. Broadly, these showed that the simple running suture (which surgeons mostly still use) is the weakest of these sutures and that some of the new ones were as strong as the core sutures. In 1996, Manske's team[35] looked at tendons repaired with circumferential sutures only, and recorded breaking strengths of up to 63 N. The multiple gripping bites of the newer circumferential sutures are not unlike core sutures in principle. Initially these new circumferential sutures were perceived as a possible alternative to elaborate core sutures rather than a way of augmenting the latter. However, the Kubota study also showed that the more material there is on the surface of the tendon, the more friction there is on mobilization, identifying an upper limit to how much one can elaborate the circumferential suture.[35]

Treatment of the Sheath: Venting of the Pulleys

In retrospect, a factor in the results achieved by the authors in the 1990s, which received no attention at the time but was, possibly, of significance, was that from the earliest of these studies, it has been routine to "vent" pulleys as necessary to allow repairs to travel through a full range of excursion, without impinging on the A2 or A4 pulleys, on passive movement of the finger before skin closure. For the senior author (D.E.), the conviction that this "made sense" followed a private conversation as a trainee in the mid-1980s at the Derby Hand Course with Dr Strickland. At the time, Dr Lister and others were quite adamant that these pulleys should remain entirely intact. Dr Strickland seemed less certain and the senior author, knowing the problems experienced personally in the emergency theater, was certain that venting was correct and necessary in many cases. Venting the sheath was not new: in the 1950s, and before, adhesions were thought necessary to achieve tendon healing, and surgeons cut windows in the sheath. Aware of the need to compensate for the tendon repair making the tendon bulkier, they cut the windows to allow a full passive range of motion of the repairs.[36,37] In the 1970s, following research by Lundborg and others, synovial fluid was believed to be the most important healer of the tendons, and surgeons moved to obsessive closure of the sheath. However, at that time and before, various investigators had pointed out that repaired and thickened flexor tendons

might not move freely in a closed sheath, and research work supported this view.[38] Others could find no evidence of any benefit from sheath closure, and many among the best results in the world were being achieved in series where the sheath had not been sutured. Consequently the enthusiasm for complete closure eventually diminished, and most surgeons now simply lay the sheath back in place without suturing it. Catching of repairs on the edges of the pulleys was another practical problem that went largely unmentioned throughout the era of complete sheath closure. In 1975, Duran and Houser had suggested partially releasing one side of any pulley on which any repair was catching. Strickland elaborated the technique and probably introduced the term "venting" the pulley, meaning cutting the side of it.[39] There was a reluctance to admit to a need to vent pulleys because, in practice, this usually entailed partial division of the A2 or A4 pulley, the complete integrity of which was believed to be of overriding importance to the mechanical efficiency of the flexor system.[40,41] This notion has its origin in a curious twist of logic: it had been recognized for a long time that when doing secondary flexor surgery, for the new flexor to achieve its mechanical intention of flexing the finger with power, the minimum one needed to preserve, or reconstruct, was an A2 and an A4 pulley. This tenet was carried over into primary flexor surgery as a mandate to preserve these 2 pulleys in their entirety at all costs. More recently, several research articles have shown that there is no absolute need to preserve the A2 or the A4 pulley so completely, or even at all, when most of the remainder of the sheath is intact.[42–45] The authors[9,26] confirmed the need for venting of both the A2 and the A4 pulley to achieve a full passive range of motion after tendon injury between zone 1 and the distal edge of the A2 pulley, in Tang's zones 2A and 2B. With the onset of postoperative edema, it is likely that the need for venting would be accentuated.[46] This problem also becomes more likely if more complex repairs are used, as these are likely to have greater bulk than simpler repairs. The discussion of venting was taken to its logical conclusion in 2 review articles,[13,47] the second of which analyzed the sites along the tendon sheath where tendon injury commonly occurs, and described appropriate pulley releases for each injury. This opinion is updated in more recent book chapters, and both reviews accord this process of pulley venting equal importance regarding the use of stronger repairs in increasing the margin of safety for early active mobilization.[48–50] The authors believe that the results of zone 1 primary flexor tendon surgery are equally dependent on judicious venting of the A4 pulley.[12]

BASIC CONSIDERATIONS OF REHABILITATION
Current Rehabilitation Protocols

In general, this is done in 1 of 2 ways, namely using either Kleinert rehabilitation, whereby extension of the fingers is active and flexion is passively achieved by rubber bands,[33] or Belfast rehabilitation, whereby both extension and flexion are achieved actively (see **Tables 1** and **2**).[51] Both regimes are mostly used with the fingers being protected from sudden or full movement into extension by a dorsal splint. Although there seems to be an almost infinite number of individual unit variations of the detail of the splinting shape, time of starting movement, and the ongoing regime, most commonly all fingers are protected by the splint and the splint is worn for 4 to 5 weeks, the period during which rupture of the repair is most likely. The degree of flexion of the metacarpophalangeal (MCP) joints and wrist in the splint is less than was used 25 years ago. Many have reduced the wrist flexion (from that akin to a Phalen test used then) to a straight wrist, or even the extended wrist position logically suggested by Savage many years ago.[52]

Passive mobilization, introduced by Duran and Houser in 1975 and supported by Strickland and Glogovac[39] in 1980, whereby the fingers were only mobilized passively by a therapist or the patient's other hand, is now used in most units, to help Kleinert and Belfast regimes to push for better results at the extremes of movement. This regime, used alone, is very labor (therapy) intensive, with no seeming advantage over the alternatives.

CURRENT SURGICAL PRACTICE
Timing of Primary/Delayed Primary Repair

Primary repair of the flexor tendons should be as early as possible after the injury. However, there is a body of evidence that delay of 24 to 72 hours is not followed by poorer results, and it is likely that delayed primary repair by an experienced surgeon will achieve a better result than immediate surgery by an inexperienced surgeon. Transfer of patients to specialist units and delay in investigating, or even treating, more pressing problems is acceptable practice. Although primary treatment is generally carried out within 72 hours, this surgery need not be considered an emergency, and extension of this period is considered later.

Surgical Approach

The authors approach the flexor tendons through zig-zag (modified Bruner) skin incisions, which are deepened through the subcutaneous tissue.

In zones 1 and 2 the tendon sheath has to be circumvented, and this is done with as little disruption as possible while providing sufficient exposure to examine, then repair, the injury to the tendon(s). A window of 2 to 4 mm in length is created by enlarging the primary wound in the sheath to a transverse opening across its full width, then splitting the lateral attachments of the sheath proximally, distally, or in both directions, to allow it to be folded back, exposing the tendons. Where the tendons have been cut with the finger in extension it is often unnecessary to open the sheath more than this, as the tendon injury lies directly below the original breach of the sheath. Where the tendons have been cut with the finger in flexion, the tendon injury will lie distal to the original cut in the sheath with the finger extended. The skin incision is extended and the window in the sheath is either enlarged or, if this would involve undue division of the pulley system, the sheath is opened through a second window overlying the distal end of the tendon with the finger extended. The sheath is opened in such a way as to preserve as much of the A2 and A4 pulleys as possible. However, it is often necessary to divide one lateral attachment of the A2 or A4 pulley along part of the pulley length (**Fig. 1**), either to effect repair of the tendons or to allow the repair to glide freely through a full range of motion without snagging on the edge of a pulley, because a flexor tendon repair is inevitably of greater diameter than the original tendon, and the uninjured tendons already fit very tightly within the sheath. Fortunately the A2 pulley is of sufficient length that one-third, or slightly more, of its length can be released laterally when necessary without resulting dysfunction. The whole A4 pulley can be released laterally, without tendon bowstringing,

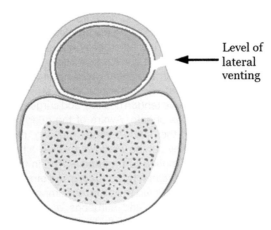

Level of lateral venting

Fig. 1. The site at which the lateral venting of the A2 pulley is made.

provided a sufficient part of the A3 and C pulleys have been retained.

Core and Peripheral Suture Methods for End-to-End Profundus Tendon Repairs

Over the last 20 years, surgeons have been bombarded with different methods of core and circumferential suturing. Many units still use a 2-strand core suture, although some have changed to, at least, a 4-strand suture (see **Table 1**). Of these, the authors find the very simple technique of inserting two 2-strand Kirchmayr/Kessler sutures in planes at right angles to each other, as recommended by Smith and Evans,[29] the simplest of these (**Fig. 2**). When a continuous suture is used to create 4 strands across the tendon junction, there remains a question as to whether all 4 strands are bearing load during movement of the repair,

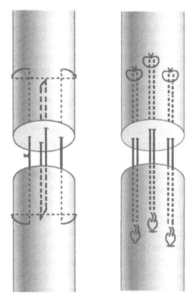

Smith and Evans (2001)
(4-strand Kessler)

Tang (1994)
(Triple Tsuge)

Fig. 2. Two core suture methods used to repair flexor digitorum profundus and some flexor digitorum superficialis tendons in fingers, and flexor pollicis longus tendons. The 4-strand core suture (*left*) advocated by Smith and Evans[29] is inserted by 2 separate groups of Kirchmayr/Kessler configuration 2-strand repair. The first suture is a conventional Kirchmayr/Kessler 2-strand repair. Before tying the knot of the first suture, another and separate Kirchmayr/Kessler suture is inserted into both ends of the tendon in the plane at right angles to the first suture. Both 2-strand Kessler suture configurations are knotted separately with a single knot for each. The 6-strand repair (*right*) is triple Tsuge sutures with looped nylon inserted equidistantly around the circumference of the tendon, as advocated by Tang and colleagues.[18]

particularly when braided sutures are used or attempts are made to lock each pass of the suture through the tendon. The Tang (triple-Tsuge) suture technique, using a looped nylon suture, is the simplest and quickest means of achieving a 6-strand core suture, at the same time obviating a circumferential suture (**Fig. 2**).[18] The authors believe this suture to be considerably simpler than the traditional "core and circumferential" combinations in routine use in Western countries. When using a 4-strand core suture the authors have reverted to a simple running circumferential suture, after using one of Silfverskiöld's circumferential sutures[30] for a time and coming to a realization that this suture is difficult to use for most training surgeons, particularly on the posterior aspect of the repair.

Repair of Profundus Tendon Close to its Insertion (Zone 1a)

The classic method of attachment of the flexor digitorum profundus (FDP) tendon to the distal phalanx with a suture passed through 1, or 2, bone holes and tied over a button at the end of the finger, or, more commonly, on the nail, works without problems in most instances. The first attempt to be rid of the button was suggested in 1965 by Pulvertaft. Various methods of avoiding the button have been devised more recently.[53] As all seem to have worked for their innovators, the argument over which is "the best" is probably futile. More pertinent is which is easiest, cheapest, and has fewest side effects: the authors prefer their own version (see **Fig. 3**)![54] Where the profundus tendon has been divided within 0.5 to 1 cm of its insertion, many surgeons are happy to excise the distal part under the assumption that the finger compensates for the slight profundus shortening. The authors see no reason to do this, and simply pass the 2 core sutures through the distal tendon segment then attach them to bone, apposing tendon to tendon and retaining the full length of the profundus.

Repair of the Retracted Tendons

Proximal retraction of the tendons from the proximal part of the finger under the A2 pulley is common. If the tendon end cannot be retrieved quickly with a fine arterial forceps passed proximally into the flexor sheath from the finger wound to grip the FDP tendon, a process that may be aided by milking the tendon from the forearm to the base of the finger with the wrist and MCP joints flexed, this should be quickly abandoned. The mid-palm is then opened, and a fine pediatric plastic tube passed distally will either carry the tendons with it to the finger wound or can be passed through

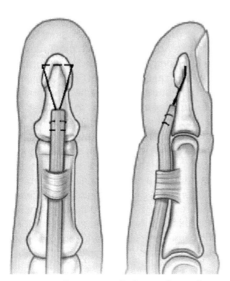

Fig. 3. The "no-button" technique of attachment of the tendon suture to the distal phalanx described by Sood and Elliot.[54] A 3/0 or 4/0 Prolene suture is attached to the distal tendon using the Kirchmayr/Kessler suture configuration. The 2 suture ends are then passed through 2 large-bore hypodermic needles inserted through a fish-mouth fingertip incision down the sides of the distal phalanx into the flexor tendon sheath at the normal tendon attachment to the phalanx. One suture end is then passed through a hole drilled in the tuft of the distal phalanx with a 1.1-mm K-wire, and the 2 suture ends are tied on the "blind" side of the finger.

the sheath to the finger wound, then sutured side-to-side to the tendons in the palm.[55] Tension on the distal end of the tube will then draw the proximal tendons out of the finger wound. The advancing profundus tendon will carry the superficialis tendon along with it.

Frayed and Diagonally Divided Profundus Tendon Ends

Trimming of frayed and/or diagonally divided tendon ends to make repair easier and/or neater should be avoided if possible, as any degree of shortening of the flexor tendons risks creating a finger that cannot extend fully at the 2 interphalangeal joints. This statement would be contested by many and the line drawn at resection of, possibly, 0.5 cm or 1 cm. A problem of trimming ragged tendon ends is that the fraying usually extends back into the tendon ends by 0.5 to 1 cm, and resection is unlikely to be less than 1 cm. Flexion of both of the interphalangeal joints in a finger synchronously, as usually occurs in these circumstances, creates a troublesome "hook finger," which usually causes more problems than are

seen when only one of the interphalangeal joints cannot extend fully. Should tendon trimming lead to a hook finger, it will almost invariably cause the patient inconvenience. Particularly if the finger is insensate following concomitant nerve injuries, it is dangerous to a machine operator. The problem should be recognized at primary surgery and rectified by tendon lengthening using Le Viet tendon lengthening in the forearm muscles,[56] or conventional tendon lengthening at the wrist for more extreme hooking of the fingers.

Superficialis Tendon Repair

Fifty years ago Kleinert and Verdan showed that it was possible and preferable to repair both flexor tendons at primary surgery, and so surgeons carry on repairing both flexor tendons under nearly every circumstance. Repair of the flexor digitorum superficialis (FDS) can be difficult in certain circumstances, as it is not always tubular. At its bifurcation the FDS is flat, it surrounds the profundus tendon, and it lies under the A2 pulley, in the so-called Tang zone 2C,[26] making any repair likely to stick. If only half the tendon is intact, the other half can be excised proximally and distally. Proximally this is taken back to the palm, and the cut half of the FDS removed obliquely so it cannot snag on the A1 or proximal A2 pulley edges. Distally it only needs be cut back to where the FDS lies flat behind the profundus tendon.

The authors' method of repair of the FDS depends on whether it has been cut in a flat or a round part of the tendon. (1) When the FDS injury is close to its insertions to the middle phalanx or in the distal part of the chiasma, usually each half is sutured separately using a horizontal mattress suture with the knot outwards (laterally) and, thus, away from the profundus tendon. This approach creates a 4-strand repair, although the authors were doing this long before 4-strand repairs were topical. (2) Proximal to the chiasma, where the tendon is anterior to the FDP and still flat, traditionally the authors have sutured this with a 4/0 Prolene 2-strand Kessler plus 5/0 or 6/0 circumferential nylon or Prolene. However, one must be aware that this repair would be under the A2 pulley, so the necessary pulley resection must be sufficient to allow suturing of the FDP tendon, to enable a full range of motion passively without snagging. It is this situation, a zone 2C repair under the A2 pulley, of which Tang wrote of suturing the FDP only.[57] The authors examined their 2C repairs at that time and did not find a problem for simple lacerations,[9] but were aware of a definite problem of the swollen tendon repairs jamming under the A2 pulley if the greater edema likely in more traumatic injuries was not appreciated and a switch to FDP suturing only was not made. In such situations, this switch was usually made by the senior author, either in person or on the telephone, and most flexor repairs at the time were being done by senior fellows who were aware of the writings of Tang and of the senior author. Perhaps the "FDP suture only" policy should be given more consideration here, as it is the safest thing to do and involves less understanding by less experienced surgeons. The authors also suspect it might often be difficult to get a 4-strand or 6-strand repair into this flat tendon, then follow it with a circumferential suture. (3) Once the tendon injury is more proximal and the FDS is thickening up, and moving to be situated under the proximal A2 and/or A1 pulley, putting whatever sutures one favors into both tendons becomes less of a problem.

Repair Under the A2 Pulley

Where both slips of the FDS are divided, the profundus is also likely to be divided, a situation that gives rise to another problem. In the 1970s, Boyes had pointed out the problem of repairs sticking under the A2 pulley, which is the tightest part of the sheath; more recently, Tang re-examined this problem and showed better results when only the profundus was repaired for injuries under the A2 pulley.[57] As mentioned earlier, the authors were unable to agree with this for simple flexor tendon divisions in a later study.[9] However, this single tendon repair is undoubtedly correct in more complex injuries of the distal palm and proximal part of the fingers, such as crush injuries at this level, distally based flaps on the distal palm, replants/revascularizations, and multifinger injuries. During the last 20 years, the senior author has treated 10 patients with such injuries of the distal palm or bases of the fingers in whom both tendons were repaired at primary surgery and in whom it was necessary to perform a tenolysis subsequently. In all cases, the 2 flexor tendons were so edematous that they were up to double their normal diameter and, as a consequence, completely jammed under the A2 pulley, with no possibility of mobilization after the first procedure. All required removal of the FDS tendon completely to allow any movement of the profundus tendon under the A2 pulley. Tang's single tendon repair at primary surgery would have avoided this secondary surgery, and the senior author has come to realize that this is the safest policy for these particular injuries under all circumstances, particularly in the hands of less experienced surgeons. The authors now only repair the profundus tendon in any injury in this area that is likely to produce significant edema.

Repair Under the A4 Pulley

Injuries under the A4 pulley, in either zone 1 or zone 2, are less problematic, as the authors consider it acceptable to completely divide the A4 pulley if necessary, provided the sheath proximally is mostly intact.[9,12,13,42,45]

Repair in the Carpal Tunnel

Although severe injuries in the carpal tunnel (zone 4), are rarer, the same problem arises for multiple tendon repairs as for under the A2 pulley, namely of lack of space. If multiple tendons are divided in zone 4, the authors repair only the profundus tendons. These repairs are likely to be particularly bulky in patients who suffer glass lacerations of several tendons that penetrate the skin of the wrist in such a way that the shard of glass passes distally into the carpal tunnel, as these tendon divisions are likely to be frayed and diagonal.

Repair of the FPL Tendon

The principles and techniques of repair of the FPL tendon are essentially the same as those of the finger profundus tendons, other than specific actions to overcome the difficulties encountered as a result of retraction of the FPL,[27,58] this may cause problems of retraction of the tendon into the carpal tunnel after division in the proximal thumb, requiring passage back through the thenar muscles, sometimes with the aid of a fine pediatric tube (see Repair of the Retracted Tendons), and difficulties of suture of the tendon ends without tendon lengthening[56] and with increased risk of rupture.[31]

Preferred Rehabilitation Protocol

In 1989, the hand surgeons in Belfast mobilized routine zone 2 flexor tendon repairs in a Kleinert traction splint, but without the elastic bands; that is, actively moving the fingers when flexing as well as when extending.[51] Many before had never used rubber bands, or had tried to get rid of them. The desire to be free of the rubber bands had been prevalent for years, largely because of the problems arising from the flexed resting position of the proximal interphalangeal joints in Kleinert traction and, also, because of difficulties in managing Kleinert traction. It was also realized that many patients never used the rubber bands to passively flex, but simply flexed their fingers actively. The senior author repeated the Belfast experiment.[7,59] Using a 2-strand core suture and a simple circumferential suture followed by rehabilitation with a modification (**Figs. 4** and **5, Table 3**) of the Belfast regimen (early active finger motion), a rupture rate of 5% for zone 1 injuries and 4%

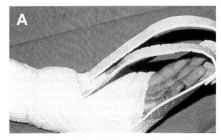
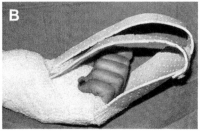

Fig. 4. Illustration of the original Billericay/Chelmsford variation of the Belfast splint, with (*A*) the fingers resting in extension and (*B*) the fingers actively flexing.

for zone 2 injuries was achieved in 440 patients with 728 complete tendon divisions in 526 fingers.[10] Others reported a similar rupture rate using variants of the Belfast regime (see **Table 1**).[60,61] The rupture rate was similar to that reported at the time by units worldwide using the Kleinert regimen (see **Table 1**), confirming the safety of this simpler and less expensive method of rehabilitation. However, the authors also reached the conclusions that (1) argument over which of the two was the better was probably unproductive, and that (2) the problem of rupture had not been solved for the fingers.

MANAGEMENT UNDER DIFFICULT CLINICAL SITUATIONS
Delayed Presentation

Largely as a result of discovering an article written back in the 1960s,[62] the significance of which was probably not appreciated at that time, the authors are now much more enthusiastic than previously with respect to delayed primary repair. This article identified the fact that delayed primary repair is possible far more often than is thought, and for far longer after the index injury. At that time, surgeons in North America were attempting to undertake the Kleinert/Verdan/Young-Harman philosophy of immediate repair and immediate mobilization. However, the hand units were still receiving patients at fairly long times after the initial

injury, as the senders were expecting them to be treated by secondary grafting in the conventional manner of that time. McFarlane and colleagues[78] tried to carry out primary repairs in 100 patients sent slowly to them, whatever the delay. Several of these patients arrived more than 12 months after the initial injury. That the flexors in 36% of 100 fingers could be repaired directly, even months after the injury, negates the assumption that delayed presentation routinely necessitates tendon grafting. With the possibility of slight tendon lengthening in the muscles without slowing the early mobilization program,[56] this figure might now be even higher. Nowadays, if a patient arrives later than 72 hours, and the finger is not infected and is mobile passively, the authors explore the finger immediately and try to repair the tendons. If the tendon ends will not quite come together, a Le Viet tendon lengthening within the muscle in the forearm is performed.[56] Although the tendon is cut, the muscle has not been, and the muscle maintains the continuity needed to allow immediate mobilization. If repair still proves impossible, then a graft can be placed with no loss of time, or a silicone rod is put in place for a staged tendon grafting procedure.

Rupture of Primary Repairs

Although concern about tendon rupture had been one of the major determinants in the evolution of

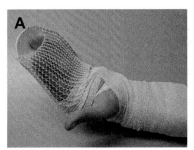
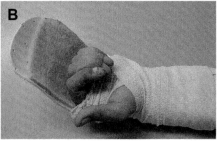

Fig. 5. Illustration of the current Billericay/Chelmsford variation of the Belfast splint, with (*A*) the fingers resting in extension and (*B*) the fingers actively flexing.

Table 3
The current St Andrews rehabilitation regime

	2012 St Andrew's Centre Early Active Mobilization Regime
Day 1	Dorsal thermoplastic splint applied Wrist straight; metacarpophalangeal joint 40° flexion; interphalangeal joints straight
Week 1	Discharged from hospital when pain controlled by simple oral analgesics, patient able to do dressings and achieving full extension to splint, and active flexion to 25% of full flexion. Instructed to carry out 10 active flexion and extension exercises per hour
Week 2	Seen by surgeons and therapists. Full extension to splint and active flexion to 50% of full flexion. Ten exercise repetitions per hour. Passive flexion exercises started
Weeks 3, 4	Seen weekly by therapists only. Full extension to the splint and progression to full range of active flexion as soon as possible (usually achieved by the end of week 3). Ten exercise repetitions per hour. Passive exercises. Ultrasound started if necessary in week 3
Week 5	Seen by surgeons and therapists. Splint removed, except at night and when risk to the hand (eg, in crowds). Wrist extension started, with fingers relaxed at first
Weeks 6, 7	Seen weekly by therapists. Progression to full range of movements of wrist and fingers
Week 8	Splint discarded completely. Passive extension exercises and dynamic extension splinting started if necessary. All but heavy activities allowed, including driving. Return to work (except heavy manual workers)
Week 10	Progressive return to heavy work by week 12

tendon suture and early postoperative mobilization throughout the last 10 years of the twentieth century, there was almost no information in the literature early in this century as to whether immediate rerepair of ruptures was successful. In 1982, Leddy stated that "the preferred treatment (of ruptures) is prompt reexploration and repair," without proof that this treatment was correct. The rupture of the tendon is most in the first month after primary repair (**Table 4**). In 2006, the authors reviewed all rupture rerepairs of zone 1 and zone 2 primary flexor tendon repairs in their unit between 1989 and 2003 to assess the outcome of immediate rerepair (**Table 5**), with a view to identifying whether this should be an invariable policy.[16] This study

Table 4
Timing of tendon ruptures after primary tendon repair

Time of Rupture (Weeks)	Number of Ruptures
<1	6
1–2	2
2–3	6
3–4	5
4–5	3
6–9	0
10	1

Data from Harris SB, Harris D, Foster AJ, et al. The aetiology of acute rupture of flexor tendon repairs in zones 1 and 2 of the fingers during early mobilization. J Hand Surg Br 1999;24:275–80.

identified that rupture rerepair, whenever possible, works adequately for all locations in zone 1 and 2 (**Table 5**) and all digits except the little finger (see later discussion).[16,79]

Certain preoperative factors require consideration before undertaking immediate rerepair and may preclude this, namely the general medical condition of the patient, advanced or very young age, a noncompliant patient, other hand abnormalities such as gross multijoint osteoarthritis, infection and/or skin breakdown in the involved finger, or a swollen and stiff finger, either because presentation is too long after the rupture, because the rupture occurs too late after the primary repair, or for other reasons. Patient refusal is most likely when an FDP tendon ruptures and proximal interphalangeal (PIP) joint flexion by an intact FDS tendon is adequate for his or her function. Occasionally, at surgery repair is impossible, owing to the friability of the tendons or because of the degree of scarring of the tendons and sheath.

The Little Finger

The authors have previously discussed technical difficulties encountered in repairing the small tendons in the little finger.[13] The small size of the digit also makes rehabilitation after primary repair more difficult. This experience was repeated in rerepairing ruptures of the primary repairs (**Table 6**).[16,79] The percentage of ruptures of primary repairs was very much greater in the little finger (46%) than in the other fingers (**Table 6**). Rerepair had a 35% chance of creating a little

Table 5
The results of immediate re-repair and successful rehabilitation of ruptures of primary flexor tendon repairs in the different zones (n = 37)

Locations	Number of Ruptures	Results of Immediate Re-repair of Ruptures			
		Excellent	Good	Fair	Poor
All fingers	37	9 (24%)	10 (27%)	5 (14%)	13 (35%)
Zone 1	5	1 (20%)	2 (40%)	0 (0%)	2 (40%)
Zone 2	32	8 (25%)	8 (25%)	5 (16%)	11 (34%)
Zone 2A	1	0	1	0	0
Zone 2B	21	5	5	4	7
Zone 2C	8	2	2	1	3
Zone 2D	2	1	0	0	1

Data from Dowd MB, Figus A, Harris SB, et al. The results of immediate re-repair of zone 1 and 2 primary flexor tendon repairs which rupture. J Hand Surg Br 2006;31:507–13; and Strickland JW, Glogovac, SV. Digital function following flexor tendon repair in Zone II: a comparison of immobilization and controlled passive motion techniques. J Hand Surg Am 1980;5:537–43.

finger that is a hindrance to grip function and a 20% chance of a second rupture. Second rupture was almost exclusively a problem of the little finger. Unfortunately, secondary surgery to the flexor tendons of this finger is no less difficult, and the only solution to the problems after primary repair is to acknowledge them and increase therapy time for these patients. The findings support a policy of no rerepair in the little finger, particularly if patient compliance or other problems have become apparent during rehabilitation. The authors believe that most ruptures of the little finger should be treated by 2-stage reconstruction, a rod being inserted into the finger as an alternative to rerepair. Rerepair of a rupture of the profundus tendon with a strong intact FDS

Table 6
Results of immediate rerepair of ruptures of primary flexor tendon repairs in zones 1 and 2 of the fingers

Results	Index	Middle	Ring	Little	Total
Excellent	2	4	1	2	9 (24%)
Good	4	3	0	3	10 (27%)
Fair	1	0	0	4	5 (14%)
Poor	1	4	1	7	13 (35%)
Second rupture	0	1	0	4	5

The results are only for the 37 fingers rehabilitated successfully out of a total of 42 fingers with tendon ruptures. Assessment was by the original Strickland criteria (1980). Rerepair was done in zones 1 in 5 fingers and in zone 2 in 32 fingers. All 5 second ruptures were in zone 2.
Data from Dowd MB, Figus A, Harris SB, et al. The results of immediate re-repair of zone 1 and 2 primary flexor tendon repairs which rupture. J Hand Surg Br 2006;31:507–13.

tendon is not recommended. Unfortunately, even when only the FDP tendon of the little finger has ruptured, doing nothing may not be an option because the FDS tendon may be absent, or too weak to provide sufficient PIP joint flexion.

The Noncompliant Patient

In 1999 we established that around 50% of the ruptures that occurred between 1989 and 1996 were in noncompliant patients.[10] Unwitting patient-related causes of rupture and bad results included some children, patients incapable of comprehending what was required of them, excessive scar formers, patients with social circumstances precluding therapy attendance, and patients with low pain thresholds. We can help these individuals more, given thought and/or adequate resources. "Uncooperative" patients include adults and children who do not comply and small children who cannot. Noncompliant adults constitute the major concern, as this injury occurs mainly in adults and does so at an age, and in a social group, where improving compliance is likely to be difficult. More time spent in therapy and psychological manipulation is the only means we have of improving the results of these patients.

The Severe Injury

Emergency referral of bad hand injuries that include flexor tendon division, or more, is inevitable for us all. We cannot redirect such injuries, but we can modify our response to them. These injuries are often added to the list of emergencies to be done by trainee surgeons, often with little expertise in this field. The consequence is inevitable, and too frequently excused as a bad result from a bad injury. These cases need the same level of senior attention as amputated fingers for replantation or high-pressure injection injuries. Given our failure to achieve normal hands after primary flexor tendon surgery routinely in even simple cases, and the passing of the earlier Louisville philosophy that the sun should never set on a cut flexor tendon, there is a case for all flexor tendon divisions being considered difficult surgery and for their being repaired by more experienced hand surgeons. This truism applies even more to complex injuries.

Multiple finger injuries present no particular problem other than the time needed to carry out the task. Pulley destruction and/or skin loss do not preclude primary repair of simple flexor tendon injuries, although the need for reconstruction of the latter may delay mobilization slightly. However, all of these situations may require the expertise of a senior surgeon, for reasons of speed and/or the reconstructive ability required. If a complex wound, sometimes with skin and subcutaneous tissue loss, is also very dirty, adequate debridement of the flexor aspect of the hand and fingers at a single operation without too much destruction of vital longitudinal structures can be difficult, or impossible. A policy of reviewing the wound in the theater 48 hours after the first exploration (policy of "48 hour look") has to be instigated. It may then become clear that flexor tendon repair is impossible and that secondary reconnection of the tendons will be necessary. Primary repair of flexor tendons in the presence of frank wound infection should not be attempted.

Most reported clinical series of acute flexor tendon repairs and rehabilitation only include simpler cases. Our knowledge of the effectiveness of current techniques of primary flexor tendon repair and rehabilitation is restricted to that gained from examination of the results of treatment of simple injuries. However, this leaves us in a position where we do not know whether the techniques suitable for simple cases should be applied to more severe injuries. More clinical articles are required, using the same assessment techniques but examining primary flexor tendon repair in adversity, that is, in association with other injuries.

Rehabilitation of More Complex Situations

The authors use exactly the same splint and Belfast regime, after simple primary flexor tendon repairs, more complex primary repairs, secondary tendon grafting, flexor tendon transfers, and revascularization/replantation, with the start of rehabilitation being delayed a few days in the latter. The authors believe that rehabilitation is not only simpler but likely to be safer and more effective if it is standardized, whenever possible, and the

therapists do not have to apply techniques they use rarely to the most difficult hands they are asked to mobilize. If a flexor tendon, or its repair, is deemed (at surgery) to be too fragile to withstand early active mobilization, it is better to replace the tendon rather than risk rupture in the immediate postoperative period. It could be argued that this regimen may be relaxed in secondary surgery, as the suture techniques are stronger than those of primary flexor tendon surgery.

SUMMARY

The authors believe that the way forward in primary flexor tendon surgery clinically is by use of strengthened but simpler sutures, appropriate venting of the pulley system, and maintaining early rehabilitation. However, there needs also be consideration of patient factors and other aspects. Perhaps surgeons have been too obsessed with strengthening of sutures in the last decades, and increasing the foreign-body suture material within the tendon may even be deleterious.[80] Research needs to continue more widely, in both the laboratory and clinical environment, until better ways of modifying adhesion of the tendon are found.

REFERENCES

1. Harmer TW. Tendon suture. Boston Med Surg J 1917;177:808–10.
2. Kulkarni M, Harris SB, Elliot D. The significance of extensor tendon tethering and dorsal joint capsule tightening after injury to the hand. J Hand Surg Br 2006;31:52–60.
3. Kirchmayr L. Zurtechnik der Sehnenaht. Zentralbl Chir 1917;44:27–52.
4. Bunnell S. Repair of tendons in the fingers and description of two new instruments. Surg Gynecol Obstet 1918;126:103–10.
5. Amadio P, An KN, Ejeskar A, et al. IFSSH Flexor Tendon Committee report. J Hand Surg Br 2005; 30:100–16.
6. Tang JB, Wu YF, Cao Y, et al. Gene therapy for tendon healing. In: Tang JB, Amadio PC, Guimberteau JC, et al, editors. Tendon surgery of the hand. Philadelphia: Elsevier Saunders; 2012. p. 59–70.
7. Elliot D, Moiemen NS, Flemming AF, et al. The rupture rate of acute flexor tendon repairs mobilized by the controlled active motion regimen. J Hand Surg Br 1994;19:607–12.
8. Yii NW, Urban M, Elliot D. A prospective study of flexor tendon repair in zone 5. J Hand Surg Br 1998;23:642–8.
9. Kwai-Ben I, Elliot D. "Venting" or partial lateral release of the A2 and A4 pulleys after repair of

zone 2 flexor tendon injuries. J Hand Surg Br 1998; 23:649–54.

10. Harris SB, Harris D, Foster AJ, et al. The aetiology of acute rupture of flexor tendon repairs in zones 1 and 2 of the fingers during early mobilization. J Hand Surg Br 1999;24:275–80.

11. Sirotakova M, Elliot D. Early active mobilization of primary repairs of the flexor pollicis longus tendon. J Hand Surg Br 1999;24:647–53.

12. Moiemen NS, Elliot D. Early active mobilization of primary flexor tendon repairs in zone 1. J Hand Surg Br 2000;25:78–84.

13. Elliot D. Primary flexor tendon repair-operative repair, pulley management and rehabilitation. J Hand Surg Br 2002;27:507–14.

14. Elliot D, Harris SB. The assessment of flexor tendon function after primary tendon repair. Hand Clin 2003;19:495–503.

15. Sirotakova M, Elliot D. Early active mobilization of primary repairs of the flexor pollicis longus tendon with two Kessler two strand core sutures and a strengthened circumferential suture. J Hand Surg Br 2004;29:531–5.

16. Dowd MB, Figus A, Harris SB, et al. The results of immediate re-repair of zone 1 and 2 primary flexor tendon repairs which rupture. J Hand Surg Br 2006;31:507–13.

17. Giesen T, Sirotakova M, Copsey AJ, et al. Flexor pollicis longus primary repair: further experience with the Tang technique and controlled active mobilisation. J Hand Surg Eur 2009;34:758–61.

18. Tang JB, Shi D, Gu YQ, et al. Double and multiple looped suture tendon repair. J Hand Surg Br 1994; 17:699–703.

19. Savage R, Risitano G. Flexor tendon repair using a "six strand" method of repair and early active mobilisation. J Hand Surg Br 1989;14:396–9.

20. Tang JB, Xie RG. Biomechanics of core and peripheral tendon repairs. In: Tang JB, Amadio PC, Guimberteau JC, et al, editors. Tendon surgery of the hand. Philadelphia: Elsevier Saunders; 2012. p. 35–48.

21. Barrie KA, Tomak SL, Cholewicki J, et al. Effect of suture locking and suture caliber on fatigue strength of flexor tendon repairs. J Hand Surg Am 2001;26:340–6.

22. Taras JS, Raphael JS, Marczyk SC, et al. Evaluation of suture caliber in flexor tendon repair. J Hand Surg Am 2001;26:1100–4.

23. Mantero R, Bertolotti P, Badoini C. Il pull-out in "no man's land" e al canale digitale nelle lesioni dei flessori (metodo personale). Riv Chir Mano 1973–1974;11:119–30.

24. Mantero R, Bertolotti P, Badoino C, et al. Revisione critica di 20 anni di esperienza sul trattamento delle lesioni dei flessori. Riv Chir Mano 1974–1975;12: 87–110.

25. Kessler I, Nissim F. Primary repair without immobilisation of flexor tendon division within the digital sheath. Acta Orthop Scand 1969;40:587–601.

26. Tang JB, Shi D. Subdivision of flexor tendon "no man's land" and different treatment methods in each sub-zone. A preliminary report. Chin Med J (Engl) 1992;105:60–8.

27. Murphy FG. Repair of laceration of flexor pollicis longus tendon. J Bone Joint Surg Am 1937;19:1121–3.

28. Urbaniak JR. Repair of the flexor pollicis longus. Hand Clin 1985;1:69–75.

29. Smith AM, Evans DM. Biomechanical assessment of a new type of flexor tendon repair. J Hand Surg Br 2001;26:217–9.

30. Silfverskiöld KL, May EJ. Flexor tendon repair in zone II with a new suture technique and an early mobilization program combining passive and active flexion. J Hand Surg Am 1994;19:53–60.

31. Kasashima T, Kato H, Minami A. Factors influencing prognosis after direct repair of the flexor pollicis longus tendon: multivariate regression model analysis. Hand Surg 2002;7:171–6.

32. Baer W, Jungwirth N, Wulle C, et al. The Mantero technique for flexor tendon repair—an alternative? Handchir Mikrochir Plast Chir 2003;35: 363–7.

33. Lister G, Kleinert HE, Kutz JE, et al. Primary flexor tendon repair followed by immediate controlled mobilisation. J Hand Surg Am 1977;2:441–51.

34. Wade PJ, Muir IF, Hutcheon LL. Primary flexor tendon repair: the mechanical limitations of the modified Kessler technique. J Hand Surg Br 1986;11:71–6.

35. Kubota H, Aoki M, Pruitt DL, et al. Mechanical properties of various circumferential tendon suture techniques. J Hand Surg Br 1996;21:474–80.

36. Mason ML. Primary and secondary tendon suture. A discussion of significance in tendon surgery. Surg Gynecol Obstet 1940;70:392–404.

37. Verdan C. La reparation immédiate des tendons fléchisseursdans le canal digital. Acta Orthop Belg 1958;24(Suppl III):15–23.

38. Tang JB, Shi D, Zhang QG. Biomechanical and histological evaluation of tendon sheath management. J Hand Surg Am 1996;21:900–8.

39. Strickland JW, Glogovac SV. Digital function following flexor tendon repair in Zone II: a comparison of immobilization and controlled passive motion techniques. J Hand Surg Am 1980;5:537–43.

40. Barton NJ. Experimental study of optimal location of flexor tendon pulleys. Plast Reconstr Surg 1969;43:125–9.

41. Idler RS, Strickland JW. The effects of pulley resection on the biomechanics of the PIP joint. J Hand Surg Am 1984;9:595.

42. Savage R. The mechanical effect of partial resection of the digital fibrous flexor sheath. J Hand Surg Br 1990;15:435–42.

43. Tomaino M, Mitsionis G, Basitidas J, et al. The effect of partial excision of the A2 and A4 pulleys on the biomechanics of finger flexion. J Hand Surg Br 1998;23:50–2.

44. Mitsionis G, Bastidas JA, Grewal R, et al. Feasibility of partial A2 and A4 pulley excision: effect on finger flexor tendon biomechanics. J Hand Surg Am 1999;24:310–4.

45. Franko OI, Lee NM, Finneran JJ, et al. Quantification of partial or complete A4 pulley release with FDP repair in cadaveric tendons. J Hand Surg Am 2011;36:439–45.

46. Wu YF, Zhou YL, Tang JB. Relative contribution of tissue oedema and the presence of an A2 pulley to resistance to flexor tendon movement: an in vitro and in vivo study. J Hand Surg Eur 2012; 37:310–5.

47. Tang JB. Indications, methods, postoperative motion and outcome evaluation of primary flexor tendon repairs in zone 2. J Hand Surg Eur 2007; 32:118–29.

48. Tang JB. Treatment of the flexor tendon sheath and pulleys. In: Tang JB, Amadio PC, Guimberteau JC, et al, editors. Tendon surgery of the hand. Philadelphia: Elsevier Saunders; 2012. p. 88–97.

49. Elliot D. Venting of the major pulleys. In: Tang JB, Amadio PC, Guimberteau JC, et al, editors. Tendon surgery of the hand. Philadelphia: Elsevier Saunders; 2012. p. 98–103.

50. Elliot D. Clinical primary flexor tendon repair and rehabilitation. The Chelmsford experience. In: Tang JB, Amadio PC, Guimberteau JC, et al, editors. Tendon surgery of the hand. Philadelphia: Elsevier Saunders; 2012. p. 125–32.

51. Small JO, Brennen MD, Colville J. Early active mobilisation following flexor tendon repair in zone 2. J Hand Surg Br 1989;14:383–91.

52. Savage R. The influence of wrist position on the minimum force required for active movement of the interphalangeal joints. J Hand Surg Br 1988; 13:262–8.

53. Wilson S, Sammut D. Flexor tendon graft attachment: a review of methods and a newly modified tendon graft attachment. J Hand Surg Br 2003; 28:116–20.

54. Sood MK, Elliot D. A new technique of attachment of flexor tendons to the distal phalanx without a button tie-over. J Hand Surg Br 1996;21: 629–32.

55. Sourmelis SG, McGrouther DA. Retrieval of the retracted flexor tendon. J Hand Surg Br 1987;12: 109–11.

56. Le Viet D. Flexor tendon lengthening by tenotomy at the musculotendinous junction. Ann Plast Surg 1986;17:239–46.

57. Tang JB. Flexor tendon repair in zone 2C. J Hand Surg Br 1994;19:72–5.

58. Elliot D. Primary repair of the flexor pollicis longus tendon. In: Tang JB, Amadio PC, Guimberteau JC, et al, editors. Tendon surgery of the hand. Philadelphia: Elsevier Saunders; 2012. p. 186–93.

59. Bainbridge LC, Robertson C, Gillies D, et al. A comparison of post-operative mobilization of flexor tendon repairs with "passive flexion-active extension" and "controlled active motion" techniques. J Hand Surg Br 1994;19:517–21.

60. Cullen KW, Tolhurst P, Lang D, et al. Flexor tendon repair in zone 2 followed by controlled active mobilisation. J Hand Surg Br 1989;14:392–5.

61. Baktir A, Türk CY, Kabak S, et al. Flexor tendon repair in zone 2 followed by early active mobilization. J Hand Surg Br 1996;21:624–8.

62. Peck FH, Bucher CA, Watson SJ, et al. An audit of flexor tendon injuries in zone II and its influence on management. J Hand Ther 1996;9:306–8.

63. Olivier LC, Assenmacher S, Kendoff D, et al. Results of flexor tendon repair of the hand by the motion-stable wire suture by Towfigh. Arch Orthop Trauma Surg 2001;121:212–8.

64. Klein L. Early active motion flexor tendon protocol using one splint. J Hand Ther 2003;16:199–206.

65. Golash A, Kay A, Warner JG, et al. Efficacy of ADCON-T/N after primary flexor tendon repair in Zone II: a controlled clinical trial. J Hand Surg Br 2003;28:113–5.

66. Peck FH, Kennedy SM, Watson JS, et al. An evaluation of the influence of practitioner-led hand clinics on rupture rates following primary tendon repair in the hand. Br J Plast Surg 2004;57:45–9.

67. Su BW, Solomons M, Lubbers L, et al. Device for zone-II flexor tendon repair. A multicenter, randomized, blinded, clinical trial. J Bone Joint Surg Am 2005;87:923–35.

68. Hung LK, Pang KW, Yeung PL, et al. Active mobilisation after flexor tendon repair: comparison of results following injuries in zone 2 and other zones. J Orthop Surg (Hong Kong) 2005;13: 158–63.

69. Caulfield RH, Maleki-Tabrizi A, Patel H, et al. Comparison of zones 1 to 4 flexor tendon repairs using absorbable and unabsorbable four-strand core sutures. J Hand Surg Eur 2008;33:412–7.

70. Hoffmann GL, Büchler U, Voeglin E. Clinical results of flexor tendon repair in zone II using a six-strand double-loop technique compared with a two-strand technique. J Hand Surg Eur 2008;33:418–23.

71. Al-Qattan MM, Al-Turaiki TM. Flexor tendon repair in zone 2 using a six-strand 'figure of eight' suture. J Hand Surg Eur 2009;34:322–8.

72. De Aguiar G, Chait LA, Schultz D, et al. Chemoprotection of flexor tendon repairs using botulinum toxin. Plast Reconstr Surg 2009;124:201–9.

73. Kitis PT, Buker N, Kara IG. Comparison of two methods of controlled mobilisation of repaired

flexor tendons in zone 2. Scand J Plast Reconstr Surg Hand Surg 2009;43:160–5.

74. Trumble TE, Vedder NB, Seiler JG 3rd, et al. Zone-II flexor tendon repair: a randomized prospective trial of active place-and-hold therapy compared with passive motion therapy. J Bone Joint Surg Am 2010;92:1381–9.

75. Georgescu AV, Matei IR, Capota IM, et al. Modified Brunelli pull-out technique in flexor tendon repair for zone II: a study on 58 cases. Hand (NY) 2011; 6:276–81.

76. Sandow MJ, McMahon M. Active mobilisation following single cross grasp four-strand flexor tenorrhaphy (Adelaide repair). J Hand Surg Eur 2011;36:467–75.

77. Schaller P. Repair of the flexor pollicis longus tendon with the motion-stable Mantero technique. Scand J Plast Reconstr Surg Hand Surg 2010;44:163–6.

78. McFarlane RM, Lamon R, Jarvis G. Flexor tendon injuries within the finger. A study of the results of tendon suture and tendon graft. J Trauma 1968;8: 987–1003.

79. Elliot D. Treatment of rupture of primary flexor tendon repairs. In: Tang JB, Amadio PC, Guimberteau JC, et al, editors. Tendon surgery of the hand. Philadelphia: Elsevier Saunders; 2012. p. 214–8.

80. Wong JK, Cerovac S, Ferguson MW, et al. The cellular effect of a single interrupted suture on tendon. J Hand Surg Br 2006;31:358–67.

Wide-awake Flexor Tendon Repair and Early Tendon Mobilization in Zones 1 and 2

Donald H. Lalonde, MD, FRCSC[a],[*], Alison L. Martin, BSc[a],[b]

KEYWORDS

- Wide awake • Intraoperative movement testing of tendon repair • Rupture • Tenolysis
- Early active movement • Finger epinephrine

KEY POINTS

- Pain-free unsedated patients with no tourniquet can comfortably test the flexor tendon repair with active movement before the skin is closed.
- Rupture rates can be decreased because gapping of the repair caused by sutures tied too loosely can be seen with intraoperative full flexion and extension. The gap can be repaired before the skin is closed.
- Tenolysis rates can be decreased because the surgeon can make pulley and repair adjustments to ensure that there is a full range of intraoperative active movement before the skin is closed.
- Watching the patient perform a full range of active movement without gapping during surgery makes the surgeon more comfortable to allow midrange active movement (as opposed to place and hold) after surgery.
- We now allow patients to perform protected midrange active flexion movement after surgery (interphalangeal joints 0° full extension to 45° flexion).

The wide-awake approach to flexor tendon repair has decreased our rupture and tenolysis rates, and permitted us to get consistently good results in cooperative patients. We no longer perform flexor tendon repair with the tourniquet, sedation, and muscle paralysis of general or block (Bier or axillary) anesthesia.

WIDE-AWAKE SURGERY: THE MERITS
Tourniquet is No Longer Necessary

Injection of only lidocaine with epinephrine wherever incisions will be made in the finger and hand permits deletion of the tourniquet, sedation, general anesthesia, and blocks (Bier or brachial plexus) that paralyze the muscles and negate comfortable patient cooperation with active finger full flexion and extension during the surgery. When patients are awake, they can test their flexor tendon repairs with a full range of active movement during the surgery.

Finger Epinephrine is Safe

Epinephrine in the finger is now known to be safe. Finger necrosis blamed on epinephrine before the 1950s when the epinephrine myth was created is now known to have been caused by procaine.[1] In 1957, phentolamine was invented. This alpha blocker has since been shown to reliably reverse

Conflict of interest: D.H. Lalonde, consultant for ASSI instruments. A.L. Martin, nil.
[a] Department of Surgery, Saint John Regional Hospital, Dalhousie University, 400 University Avenue, Saint John NB E2L 4L4, Canada; [b] Faculty of Medicine, Dalhousie University, Tupper Medical Building #382, 1459 Oxford Street, Halifax, Nova Scotia B3H 4R2, Canada
* Corresponding author. Saint John Regional Hospital, Dalhousie University, Hilyard Place, Suite C204, 600 Main Street, Saint John NB E2K 1J5, Canada.
E-mail address: drdonlalonde@nb.aibn.com

Hand Clin 29 (2013) 207–213
http://dx.doi.org/10.1016/j.hcl.2013.02.009
0749-0712/13/$ – see front matter © 2013 Elsevier Inc. All rights reserved.

epinephrine vasoconstriction in the human finger as an antidote at a dose of 1 mg injected in whichever volume is required to be injected wherever the epinephrine was injected.[2] Large series reporting the safe injection of finger epinephrine have been published in which phentolamine rescue has never been necessary.[3,4] There are no cases of finger necrosis even with accidental injection of high-dose 1:1000 epinephrine.[5]

Repairing Gaps Revealed with Intraoperative Active Movement Testing of the Repair Decreases Rupture Rates

The most important thing to avoid is gapping of the tendon repair, which leads to tendon rupture. After the repair, the patient is asked to flex and extend the finger completely. When a patient takes the tendon repair through a full active range of motion during the surgery, the surgeon sometimes observes a gap that occurs because the tendon suture is not tight enough. The gap can be repaired with a tighter suture to avoid rupture.[6] A series of 102 patients with intraoperative testing of wide-awake flexor tendon repairs by our group revealed 7 patients with intraoperative gapping that was repaired intraoperatively and did not rupture postoperatively. None of the 102 patients who followed proper postoperative instructions ruptured after surgery.[7]

Ensuring that There is a Full Range of Active Movement Before the Skin is Closed Decreases Tenolysis Rates

After the repair, the patient is asked to flex and extend the finger completely. If the repair does not fit through the pulleys during the surgery, it is not likely to fit through the pulleys later and will almost certainly require a tenolysis. However, intraoperative repair adjustments such as complete division of the A4 pulley or partial division of the A2 pulley, as advocated by Tang,[8] often permit conversion to a full range of movement. As an alternative, the repair can be trimmed with resection or slimmed with sutures if there is excessively bunched tendon that does not fit through pulleys. Full range of active flexion and extension should be ensured before the skin is closed so that tenolysis is less likely to be needed postoperatively.

Watching Gap-free Full Active Flexion and Extension During Surgery Facilitates Active Protected Movement After Surgery to Prevent the Repair from Getting Stuck

When the comfortable unsedated patient takes the finger through a full range of flexion and extension during the surgery (metacarpophalangeal [MP] joint full extension to 90° flexion, proximal interphalangeal [PIP] joint 0° full extension to 270° flexion, distal interphalangeal [DIP] joint 0° full extension to 90° flexion) without gapping or rupture, the surgeon is more confident and in allowing the patient to perform early midrange active protected movement (0° full extension to 45° flexion of MP, PIP, and DIP joints) with minimal risk of rupture.

ANESTHESIA TECHNIQUE
Volume and Concentration of Tumescent Local Anesthesia: Large Volume and Low Concentration Where Incisions and Dissection will be Performed

Lidocaine with epinephrine is injected everywhere the surgeon will be dissecting. This is like an extravascular Bier block that is injected only where surgery will be performed. We keep the total dose less than 7 mg/kg. If less than 50 mL is required, we use 1% lidocaine with 1:100,000 epinephrine. If 50 to 100 mL will be required (hand and forearm cases), we dilute the local with saline (50:50) to a mixture of 0.5% lidocaine with 1:200,000 epinephrine. In large forearms that need a volume of 100 to 200 mL to anesthetize a large area, we use 0.25% lidocaine with 1:400,000 epinephrine.[9]

How Much and Where to Inject Lidocaine with Epinephrine in the Finger and Palm

In the finger, the 1% lidocaine with 1:100,000 epinephrine is injected the subcutaneous fat in the middle of the base of the phalanges between both digital nerves so the bevel of the needle does not lacerate the fascicles.[10,11] In the proximal and middle palmar phalanges, 2 mL are injected. In the distal phalanx, 1 mL is injected.

We routinely inject 10 to 15 mL in the palm wherever dissection will be performed.

Tips to Minimize the Pain of the Local Anesthesia Injection into the Finger and Hand

- Buffer the lidocaine with epinephrine with 1 mL of 8.4% bicarbonate for each 10 mL of 1% lidocaine with epinephrine[12] (this takes the pH from 4.7 to 7.4).[13]
- Use a 27-gauge needle, instead of 25 gauge, so that it hurts less going in. Smaller gauge needles also force you to slow the injection down, which makes it less painful.
- Try to insert the needle perpendicular to the skin for less pain.[14]
- Do not inject intradermally; it hurts more. Inject 0.5 mL into the fat under the skin,

then pause until the patient tells you all that the sting is gone.

- Slowly inject at least the first 5 to 10 mL in the hand or forearm before moving the needle.
- Inject in the most proximal area that is likely to be dissected. Wait 15 to 20 minutes before injecting distally so the distal nerves have time to be blocked (**Figs. 1–4**).
- Always have at least 10 mm of local ahead of the needle so that the needle is advanced into only numb areas.
- Use more local than is expected to be needed in the hand and forearm. Patients never complain about being too numb, but they will remember you for not numbing them enough. However, do not use more than 2 mL per phalanx in the fingers to avoid too much compartment pressure.
- Blow slow before you go, blow slow before you go; repeat this mentally as you inject.
- Ask patients to tell you if they feel any pain during the injections; you will only improve your score (the number of times they feel pain during the injection process).[15]

Preoperative Planning of Local Anesthetic Injection

The patient can be injected outside of the operating room so that the epinephrine has 20 to 30 minutes or more to produce optimal vasoconstriction. The patient should be lying down for the injection because the occasional patient becomes vasovagal and possibly faints, even lying down. Patients may say that they are not feeling well or

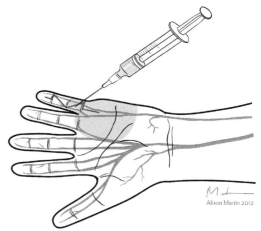

Fig. 2. Between 15 and 30 minutes after the first injection, the digital nerves are blocked and the patient des not feel the next 3 injections. Two milliliters of 1% lidocaine with 1:100,000 epinephrine buffered with 10:1 8.4% bicarbonate are injected into the fat under the skin just past the palmar digital crease between the two digital nerves. The patient does not feel this injection if the injection in **Fig. 1** has had time to work.

feel nauseated, or they may get pale between the eyes; these are symptoms and signs that they will faint. Immediately flex the hips and knees to get more blood to the brain. Then the head of the bed can be lowered in the Trendelenburg position and the pillow removed from under the patient's head to further improve blood flow to the brain.

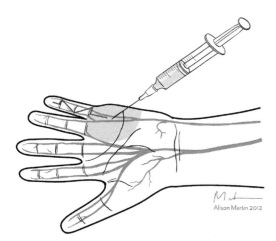

Fig. 1. Between 10 and 15 mL of 1% lidocaine with 1:100,000 epinephrine buffered with 10:1 8.4% bicarbonate are injected with a 27-gauge needle in the palm more proximal than the most proximal incision possible. The local is injected slowly just under the skin in the fat without moving the needle.

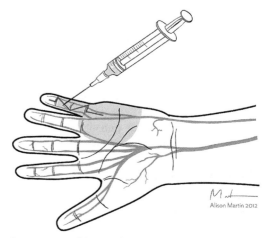

Fig. 3. Two milliliters of 1% lidocaine with 1:100,000 epinephrine buffered with 10:1 8.4% bicarbonate are then injected into the fat under the skin just past digital crease of the PIP joint between the two digital nerves. The patient does not feel this injection if the injection in **Fig. 1** has had time to work.

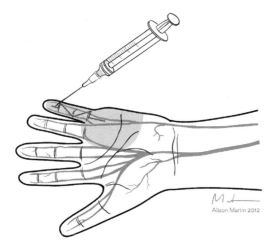

Fig. 4. One milliliter of 1% lidocaine with 1:100,000 epinephrine buffered with 10:1 8.4% bicarbonate is then injected into the fat under the skin just past digital crease of the DIP joint between the two digital nerves. The patient does not feel this injection if the injection in **Fig. 1** has had time to work.

After injection, patients should be warned that they may get a shaky feeling, as though they have had too much coffee, because of the adrenaline. They should be told that they are not allergic to it, that it is a normal reaction to the injected hormone, and that the shaky feeling will pass in 15 to 30 minutes. The half-life of epinephrine in plasma is only 1.7 minutes.[16]

Prep and Patient Positioning

During the surgery, patients can lay on their back or side, whichever is comfortable, because there is no anesthetic equipment in the way. They are allowed to watch the surgery, or parts of it, as they wish. They should wear a mask if they are speaking toward the wound. Patients with anesthetized fingers lose their proprioceptive sense and you may have to ask them to look at their fingers to get them to actively flex and extend to test the tendon repair after sutures. Most patients do not mind this, and many are interested in seeing their surgery.

SURGICAL TECHNIQUE

Wide-awake flexor tendon repair is about the anesthesia, not about the surgery. Surgeons can use whichever technique they are most comfortable with. However, the author outlines his preferred technique in this article.

Incisions and Hemostasis

Bruner or rectangular incisions with laterally based flaps decrease the risk of tendon exposure if the

wounds should come apart. The pulp of the finger tip can be cut down the center to the middle of the distal phalanx, and the scissors used to spread the soft tissues parallel to the nerves in the center of the finger over the insertion of the flexor digitorum profundus (FDP) from proximal to distal to avoid nerve damage. If the surgeon stays in the middle and uses scissors to spread the two nerve bundles apart, nerve damage is minimized. It is like taking your hand and pushing it up from the trunk to the leaves between 2 bushes in your garden. The nerves are pushed and stretched aside like the branches of the bushes.

There will be bleeding when the skin is cut, unlike when a tourniquet is used. However, by the time the skin flaps are sewn back to the finger dorsum with 4-0 nylon sutures, most of the bleeding will have stopped. We no longer use cautery, because the little bleeders stop spontaneously (or occasionally with a hemostat on bigger vessels for a few minutes). A significant reward for using no tourniquet is that there is no rebound bleeding at the end of the surgery, and the field is dry when the skin is closed. The other major reward is the avoidance of patient uncooperativeness with even light sedation, muscle paralyzing blocks (Bier and plexus), and general anesthesia.

Exposing the Sheath and Sheathotomies

The sheath is exposed from where the tendon can be seen though it proximally to where the distal tendon can be seen through the sheath distally (**Fig. 5**). A small transverse incision is then made in the sheath over the distal end of the proximal tendon. The tendon is pushed like a rope distally with 2 pairs of Adson forceps through the sheathotomy. In this way, the distal end of the tendon

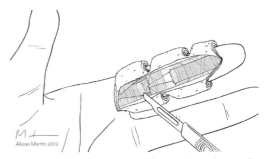

Fig. 5. The sheath is exposed from where the tendon can be seen though it proximally to where the distal tendon can be seen through the sheath distally, and a 1-cm bite of tendon is used to suture. The laterally based flaps have been sewn back to the dorsal skin and the bleeding dries by itself without cautery. A sheathotomy incision is made just proximal to the visible proximal end of the cut tendon so it can be pushed forward.

is not crushed by a hemostat or forceps that might be used to pull the tendon distally in the sheath. The tendon end that needs to heal should not be further traumatized with surgical manipulation. The FDP also finds its way more easily through the decussation of flexor digitorum superficialis (FDS) if it is pushed distally rather than retrieved with a red rubber catheter, which could take it outside the FDS decussation. The tendon is pushed sufficiently that the tendon repair can be performed with no tension. It is then held in place with needles in the sheath (**Figs. 6** and **7**).

If the Patient is Pulling Against the Surgeon

When the surgeon is trying to retrieve the proximal tendon, the patient may pull on the tendon by powering the flexors, making it difficult to get the tendon out to length. This problem is easily overcome in most patients by first asking them to relax. If that does not work, ask them to extend their fingers, which will reflexly relax their flexor muscles. The tendon is then brought out to length and held in the sheath with a needle.

Getting a 1-cm Bite of Tendon

Tang and colleagues[17,18] showed that the ideal tendon bite should be approximately 1 cm in length. To decrease the pulley and sheath division, transverse sheathotomies are made 1 cm from where the repair is to be performed to allow the needle to enter the tendon inside the sheath. This is a safe maneuver because the patient will be asked to move the tendon after each core suture to ensure that the needle has not captured part of the sheath (**Fig. 8**).

Sutures

Two locking 3-0 or 4-0 Kessler core suture repairs (4-strand repair) with Ethibond (noncutting needle)

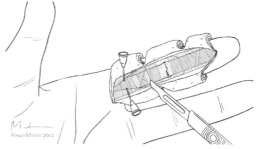

Fig. 7. A second sheathotomy is made proximally in the sheath 1 cm from the tendon ends. It is through this sheathotomy that the needle and thread are inserted to enter the tendon inside the sheath. A third sheathotomy is made similarly 1 cm distal to the repair site for distal needle and suture insertion.

are used with a running 6-0 nylon epitenon suture.[19] If the repair is not in the sheath area, no epitenon suture is required.

Intraoperative Testing of the Flexor Tendon Repair

This may be the most important part of the operation. After each core suture and after the epitenon suture, the patient is asked to completely flex and extend all fingers, including the operated digits. They may have to look at the fingers to accomplish this because the local anesthesia obliterates proprioception. The wounds can be covered with gauze if the patients are uneasy about seeing their open wounds.

If active full range of flexion and extension creates a gap in the repair, the suture was not placed tightly enough and needs to be replaced with a suture with proper tension. In the days

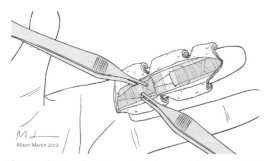

Fig. 6. The tendon is pushed forward by alternately grasping it with 2 Adson forceps through the proximal sheathotomy wound until the tendon ends are touching with less than no tension (pushing against each other so they bulge together).

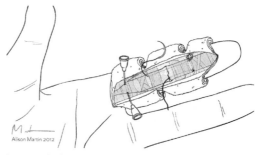

Fig. 8. A locking Kessler suture (Kessler with an extra bite to lock the suture to prevent it from sliding) is used as the first of 2 core sutures. Full active flexion and extension is then performed by the wide-awake patient after each core suture and after the epitenon suture to ensure that the suture was tight enough to avoid gapping, and to ensure that the repair moves easily through the pulleys.

before repairs were tested, these would likely have gone on to rupture.

If the repair does not fit through the pulleys, we completely resect the A4 pulley if required, and resect up to half of the A2 pulley as advocated by Tang.[8,20] As an alternative, we trim the repair or add sutures. The main thing is that the patient has a full range of flexion and extension before the skin is closed.

POSTOPERATIVE CARE AND REHABILITATION
The First 2 to 4 Days Postsurgery

We keep the hand elevated and immobile in an orthosis (splint) with the wrist in comfortable extension. The MP joint is flexed to 80° to 90°, and the PIP and DIP joints are extended for the first 2 to 4 days postsurgery. Collagen formation does not start until day 3, so serious adhesions are not likely to start before then. In addition, if patients move immediately after surgery, they may bleed inside the wound and that blood will add to the scar tissue. Also, the finger and tendons will be swollen and have more friction as they try to move in the sheath in the first 3 days. Elevation and immobilization decrease bleeding and swelling in the first days after surgery.

Days 3 to 21 Postsurgery

We follow a regime similar to that of Tang.[8] During this period, patients focus on full active extension of the interphalangeal joints with the MP joints flexed. They passively warm up the MP, PIP, and DIP joints to decrease friction and work of the tendons before starting active movement. We allow midrange active movement. This means we let them make a half a fist: 45° flexion of each of the MP, PIP, and DIP joints active flexion of the fingers. We do not allow full flexion of the PIP and DIP joints because this would increase the friction across the repair as well as risk the repair fetching on the edge of a fully flexed pulley. The lack of active movement, the friction of full flexion, and the risk of tension of the repair on the edge of a pulley in full flexion are the reasons we have abandoned the full fist form of place-and-hold form rehabilitation currently popular in North America, and replaced it with the midrange active protocol currently popular in the United Kingdom and China.

We tell patients: "You can move it but you can't use it." We get them to move both hands at the same time and look from one to the other to mimic mirror therapy. We continue to keep the finger splinted with the wrist in comfortable extension, the MP joint flexed to 80° to 90°, and the interphalangeal joint extended.

Films of the surgery and postoperative orthoses are linked to Refs.[9,21,22]

SUMMARY

The wide-awake approach to flexor tendon repair has decreased our rupture and tenolysis rates, and permitted us to get consistently good results in cooperative patients. We are now doing midrange active movement after surgery. We no longer perform flexor tendon repair with the tourniquet, sedation, and muscle paralysis of general or block (Bier or axillary) anesthesia.

REFERENCES

1. Thomson CJ, Lalonde DH, Denkler KA, et al. A critical look at the evidence for and against elective epinephrine use in the finger. Plast Reconstr Surg 2007;119:260–6.
2. Nodwell T, Lalonde DH. How long does it take phentolamine to reverse adrenaline-induced vasoconstriction in the finger and hand? A prospective randomized blinded study: the Dalhousie Project experimental phase. Can J Plast Surg 2003;11:187–90.
3. Lalonde D, Bell M, Benoit P, et al. A multicenter prospective study of 3,110 consecutive cases of elective epinephrine use in the fingers and hand: the Dalhousie Project clinical phase. J Hand Surg Am 2005;30:1061–7.
4. Chowdhry S, Seidenstricker L, Cooney DS, et al. Do not use epinephrine in digital blocks: myth or truth? Part II. A retrospective review of 1111 cases. Plast Reconstr Surg 2010;126:2031–4.
5. Fitzcharles-Bowe C, Denkler K, Lalonde D. Finger injection with high-dose (1:1000) epinephrine: does it cause finger necrosis and should it be treated? Hand 2007;2:5–11.
6. Wu YF, Tang JB. Effects of tension across the tendon repair site on tendon gap and ultimate strength. J Hand Surg Am 2012;37:906–12.
7. Higgins A, Lalonde DH, Bell M, et al. Avoiding flexor tendon repair rupture with intraoperative total active movement examination. Plast Reconstr Surg 2010; 126:941–5.
8. Tang JB. Indications, methods, postoperative motion and outcome evaluation of primary flexor tendon repairs in Zone 2. J Hand Surg Eur 2007; 32:118–29.
9. Mustoe TA, Buck DW, Lalonde DH. The safe management of anesthesia, sedation and pain in plastic surgery. Plast Reconstr Surg 2010;126: 165e–76e.
10. Thomson CJ, Lalonde DH. Randomized double-blind comparison of duration of anesthesia among three commonly used agents in digital nerve block. Plast Reconstr Surg 2006;118:429–32.

11. Williams JG, Lalonde DH. Randomized comparison of the single-injection volar subcutaneous block and the two-injection dorsal block for digital anesthesia. Plast Reconstr Surg 2006;118:1195–200.

12. Cepeda MS, Tzortzopoulou A, Thackrey M, et al. Adjusting the pH of lidocaine for reducing pain on injection. Cochrane Database Syst Rev 2010;(8). CD006581.

13. Frank SG, Lalonde DH. How acidic is the lidocaine we are injecting, and how much bicarbonate should we add? Can J Plast Surg 2012;20:71–3.

14. Martires K, Bordeaux J. Reducing the pain of lidocaine administration by controlling angle of injection. J Am Acad Dermatol 2011;64(Suppl 1): AB167.

15. Lalonde DH. "Hole-in-one" local anesthesia for wide awake carpal tunnel surgery. Plast Reconstr Surg 2010;126:1642–4.

16. Rosen SG, Linares OA, Sanfield J, et al. Epinephrine kinetics in humans: radiotracer methodology. J Clin Endocrinol Metab 1989;69:753–61.

17. Tang JB, Zhang Y, Cao Y, et al. Core suture purchase affects strength of tendon repairs. J Hand Surg Am 2005;30:1262–6.

18. Cao Y, Zhu B, Xie RG, et al. Influence of core suture purchase length on strength of four-strand tendon repairs. J Hand Surg Am 2006;31:107–12.

19. Lalonde DH. An evidence-based approach to flexor tendon laceration repair. Plast Reconstr Surg 2011; 127:885–90.

20. Tang JB. Clinical outcomes associated with flexor tendon repair. Hand Clin 2005;21:199–210.

21. Lalonde DH, Kozin S. Tendon disorders of the hand. Plast Reconstr Surg 2011;128:1e–14e.

22. Lalonde DH. Wide-awake flexor tendon repair. Plast Reconstr Surg 2009;123:623–5.

Uncommon Methods of Flexor Tendon and Tendon-Bone Repairs and Grafting

Jin Bo Tang, MD

KEYWORDS

- Flexor tendon • Late direct repair • Tendon lengthening plasty • Mini-anchor • Allograft
- Tendon-bone junction • Surgical techniques

KEY POINTS

- Although secondary tendon grafting is the standard treatment of tendon lacerations with a late presentation (a month after injury), late direct repair is possible in a small proportion of patients for whom direct approximation of the tendon ends is possible.
- Lengthening plasty of the tendon in the forearm may accommodate repair of the tendon defect or ease the tension of the end-to-end repair performed in the finger or palm.
- Newer methods, such as a mini-anchor or a reinforced suture, of attaching the flexor digitorum profundus to the distal phalanx allow early active tendon motion and replace the pull-out suture, which sometimes affects the nail and risks infection.
- Tendon allograft may become a reliable way in tendon reconstruction, provided that there are future modifications in the preservation of allografts. The author's preliminary results, with up to 5 years of follow-up, indicate no obvious clinical problems with the allografted tendons.

The common choices of repairing the flexor tendons have been stagnated in most hand units. Primary repair, whenever possible, is currently a standard practice. The technical details, surgical or postsurgical, have been evolving over the past 3 decades and remain quite diverse. When stringent surgical principles are upheld and surgeons experienced in tendon surgery perform the procedures, outcomes have improved considerably over the past decades.

Surgeons encounter injuries of varying degrees of severity and with different time periods elapsed since injury. In such cases, repair of the flexor tendons may not be as straightforward as we are normally taught.

The author presents a few methods used in selected cases over the years to address some problems. Some procedures that are presented are exploratory; they have achieved expected outcomes thus far, but they need further definition in the years to come. Indications, techniques, and outcomes of these procedures as well as clinical pitfalls are described.

LATE DIRECT REPAIR OF LACERATED TENDONS

Direct repair of the lacerated tendon is not standard practice if patients are treated a month after trauma; such patients are generally contraindicated for an end-to-end repair. The author performs secondary tendon grafting 3 months after the initial injury in most of these cases that present a month after injury. The author usually carefully examines the tension of the retracted proximal tendons and has found that in a small portion of the cases it was actually possible to pull the retracted proximal end to approximate

Department of Hand Surgery, The Hand Surgery Research Center, Affiliated Hospital of Nantong University, 20 West Temple Road, Nantong 226001, Jiangsu, China
E-mail address: jinbotang@yahoo.com

Hand Clin 29 (2013) 215–221
http://dx.doi.org/10.1016/j.hcl.2013.02.004
0749-0712/13/$ – see front matter © 2013 Elsevier Inc. All rights reserved.

the distal end. Therefore, he judged that these tendons were still candidates for direct repair without the need for tendon grafting.

Decision Making: Intraoperative Judgment

The decision whether or not to perform direct repair is not possible before surgery and patients should always be prepared for tendon grafting. There are no preoperative guidelines to help judge which cases (digits) are appropriate for such late direct repair. When multiple fingers are injured, tension can differ among fingers, making one finger possible for direct repair and others not. The index finger has more chance for such repair. Only an intraoperative test to pull the tendon ends together will tell whether late direct repair is feasible (**Figs. 1–3**), assuming the surgeon has sufficient experience with primary tendon repair. The author has treated a dozen fingers by this method and has had acceptable clinical return of function. It is judged by whether the two tendon ends can be pulled together with the finger moderately flexed; in this position, there is ample space to insert a strong core suture repair. If approximation of the two tendon ends flexes the finger very remarkably, the tension is too high, and direct repair is not considered feasible.

Surgical Techniques

Late direct tendon repair is similar to an ordinary primary repair, except that the operator

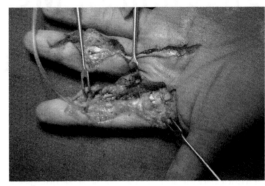

Fig. 2. A silicone guide tube was inserted to guide the proximal stump of the FDP tendon of the index finger to reach the distal stump through preserved the sheath pulleys.

consistently feels higher tension on the sutured ends, and the digits are under marked tension (manifested as moderate digital flexion) after completion of the direct repair. Strong core repair methods (6 strand or more) should be used. Peripheral sutures are attempted; however, it is usually impossible to add a running suture. Instead, interrupted stitches are added.

A strong core suture is necessary in late direct repair, which enhances repair strength and prevents gap formation, because the tension over the repair site is great. Tension across the repair site is also necessary to prevent gapping.[1,2] Intraoperative simulated active digital motion is

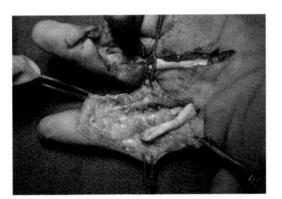

Fig. 1. A clean-cut injury to the middle part of the index and middle fingers referred for reconstruction of finger flexion 5 months after trauma. Bruner incisions were used in the index and middle fingers, for which 1-stage tendon grafting was planned. Proximal flexor digitorum profundus (FDP) tendons in both fingers were found retracted to the distal palm. The proximal FDP tendon in the index finger can be easily pulled to the proximal interphalangeal (PIP) joint level as shown in the picture. Therefore, direct repair was attempted in the index finger.

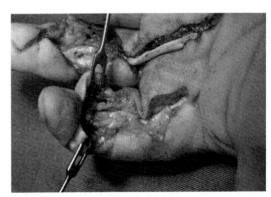

Fig. 3. The FDP tendon in the index finger could be approximately after trimming the tendon ends to refresh both stumps, and it was directly sutured with the fingers in moderate flexion. Note that tension was greater than the primarily repaired tendons that the author and his colleagues see; moderate flexion of the index was necessary to make the direct repair. In the middle finger, the tendon gliding surface of the FDP tendon was found to be abnormal; the direct repair was abandoned, and tendon grafting was performed.

performed to ensure no gapping at the repair site. The flexor digitorum superficialis (FDS) is not repaired. In the digit area, a part of the A2 pulley or the entire A4 pulley needs to be vented to permit motion of the often-thickened tendon ends. The incisions are closed and digits are in flexion after surgery (**Fig. 4**).

Postoperative Care

The finger is protected during the first 5 or 6 postoperative days, and motion is begun on day 7 to even day 10. Patients are instructed to start exercising very gently. Full extension is not achievable in most cases, even at week 5 or 6; but continuing rehabilitation to postoperative weeks 8 to 10, or even after weeks 10 to 12, is still efficient to correct the remaining extension lag. A few of the author's patients were able to improve their extension even after a few months with careful instruction. These late direct repairs generally show an intermediate degree of recovery between primary repair and secondary tendon grafting (**Fig. 5**). The cases of late direct repair should involve compliant patients only. Instructions should be given to guide gradual exercise of the muscles to correct active extension lag.

It should be noted that the cases appropriate for late direct repair are not many, and it is an unusual secondary tendon repair. The author estimates that only about 1 out of 10 to 1 out of 15 of the tendons considered for 1-stage tendon grafting may be treated alternatively. For clean-cut flexor tendons (in the digital sheath or in the palm), the operator may keep in mind the feasibility of a late direct repair. The direct repair may ultimately be possible in a small proportion of the cases whereby 2 cut tendon ends can be pulled together and tension is not extremely great, as judged

intraoperatively. This repair definitely requires a careful judgment of the operator, who ideally should be experienced in both primary repair and secondary grafting.

The additional note is about repair methods. The author used at least a 6-strand core suture repair for these late direct repairs. A 6-strand repair is used in the digital sheath area. An 8-strand or a 10-strand repair is used in the palm area; at the palm, a wider exposure is possible and larger space accommodates a greater number of core sutures.

The 10-strand core suture is a combination of a 6-strand and a 4-strand repair (**Fig. 6**), made with a normal length (7–10 mm) of suture purchase at one tendon stump and an extended purchase (12–15 mm) at the other.

TENDON LENGTHENING IN THE FOREARM

Z-plasty lengthening of the flexor tendon in the forearm is an effective way to compensate for the loss of elasticity of muscle fibers after weeks or months without tendon continuity or tension across the muscle belly. This procedure can be an adjunct to late direct tendon repair to ease tension. Le Viet[3] advocated this surgery in 1986. It is useful in 2 situations: (1) primary repair of the tendon with a defect more than 1.5 cm to 2.0 cm and (2) late direct repair of the tendon, if the tension is persistently high after surgery.

The skin incision is small, and the surgical procedure is straightforward. The tendon can be exposed in the middle or distal forearm by a 2-cm incision. Z-plasties, Z tenotomy, or accordion technique can be performed on the tendon to help increase its length. This surgery has not been used by many surgeons, but it is useful. The author prefers a forearm longitudinal incision to expose the flexor tendon and lengthening the tendon by about 1 to 2 cm. A certain amount of tension should be maintained across the lengthened site because as postoperative rehabilitation goes on, the elasticity of the muscle bellies will increase. Over-lengthening would decrease the power of finger flexion. The lengthening surgery can be performed at the time of the direct tendon repair or during the rehabilitation process (after solid healing of the directly repaired tendons, which is the author's preferred timing for this procedure).

The need for tendon lengthening in the forearm is judged according to patient function. Rehabilitation aids recovery of muscle elasticity to some extent, obviating lengthening in some cases. Some patients accept a mild extension deficit in the digit and do not want an additional surgery to lengthen the tendon.

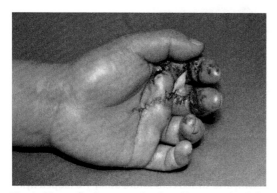

Fig. 4. Finger flexion cascade after direct repair of the flexor digitorum profundus tendon in the index finger and free tendon grafting in the middle finger.

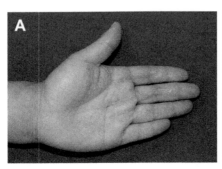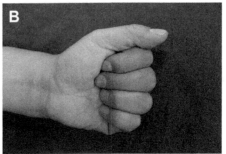

Fig. 5. One year and 6 months after surgery. (*A*) Finger extension; (*B*) finger flexion.

MICROANCHOR FOR TENDON-BONE JUNCTION

Novel methods have been reported over the last 2 decades, and have been proposed as routine methods, to replace the pull-out suture repair.[4–8] The pull-out suture has long been a standard way to achieve tendon-bone junction in the distal part of the fingers. This method is challenged by newer methods in which the nail is not violated.[4–8] Most of the recent methods have a reasonable design, although some are complex. The author has had experience with the microanchor and reinforced direct suture. Both are found comparable with the pull-out repair.

The author and his colleagues have used the Mitek microanchor (Johnson and Johnson, New Brunswick, NJ). The anchor is placed in the middle of the distal phalanx through a drill hole. The anchor should ideally be buried under the cortex of the bone. This metal anchor carries 4 suture strands (Ethibond, Johnson and Johnson) with a needle in the end of each strand. After the placement of the anchor, the 4 strands connecting to the implanted anchor are used to make multiple cross-locking stitches to increase the repair strength. These strands are tied over the tendon stump. No peripheral suture is necessary after completion (**Fig. 7**).

After surgery, the fingers undergo early active motion with a midrange active motion regime,[2] and therapy continues to postoperative weeks 6 to 8.

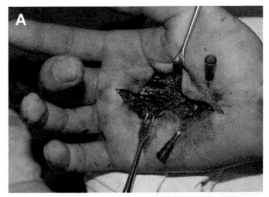

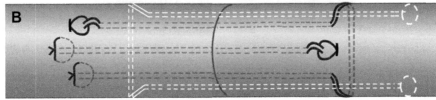

Fig. 6. (*A*) A flexor tendon laceration in the palm treated 8 months after trauma. Direct approximation of the cut ends of the FDP tendon was possible, and they were repaired with a 10-strand core suture using 4–0 looped nylon sutures, followed by interrupted peripheral suture. (*B*) The detail of the 10-strand repair: one 6-strand repair plus a U-shaped, 4-strand repair made with asymmetrical suture purchase length (7–10 mm for one and 12–15 mm for another). The repair was smooth after completion.

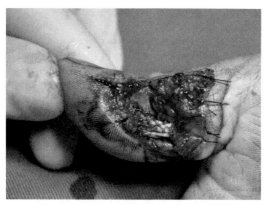

Fig. 7. A flexor pollicis longus tendon was repaired with a Mitek anchor. Note the multiple cross-stitch sutures added to the tendon stump to connect it to the anchor.

STRONG REINFORCED SUTURE FOR TENDON-BONE JUNCTION
Indications, Techniques, and Postoperative Motion

In the author's unit, a microanchor is used to achieve tendon-bone junction if the distal stump is very short. If the distal flexor digitorum profundus (FDP) tendon stump is about 1 cm, it is possible to place the grafted tendon between 2 bundles of the FDP tendon. The graft and residual parts of the FDP tendon can be sutured together with multiple reinforced sutures using 3–0 or 4–0 Ethibond or nylon sutures (**Fig. 8**).

This tendon-tendon method usually makes a strong tendon-bone junction. Although the suture site is usually bulky, the tendon does not

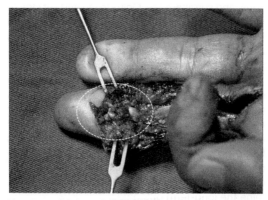

Fig. 8. Multiple reinforced sutures of the residual distal tendon stump with the grafted tendons in tendon grafting reconstruction. This repair provides a bulky yet strong tendon junction. Because there is little gliding at the distal part of the FDP tendon, this bulky repair does not affect tendon motion and joint flexion.

glide there because it is beyond the distal interphalangeal (DIP) joint. Thus, the repair would not interfere with digital flexion. The fingers undergo a rehabilitation regime similar to that used after primary repair, although generally less aggressive. Full active finger flexion is not started during the first 3 weeks. Instead, midrange active flexion is prescribed, and passive DIP joint flexion is stressed.

Microanchor Repair Versus Reinforced Suture Repair

In recent years, the author and his colleagues have rarely used a pull-out suture repair. Instead, they have been more likely to use a microanchor or a reinforced suture repair for either a distal zone 1 injury or attachment of the grafted tendon. They have not yet encountered any ruptures of this repair. In contrast, because fixation of avulsed bone after mallet finger (extensor) injury with a microanchor has caused complications, such as protrusion of the anchor, they have abandoned that approach for mallet fingers. They have not found protrusion of the anchor after distal zone 1 flexor tendon repair. The author uses a reinforced suture to achieve a tendon-bone junction in tendon grafting in the fingers and uses a microanchor when no sufficient distal stump is available. A drawback for a microanchor repair is its complexity; however, it is evolving.

TENDON ALLOGRAFT

Tendon autograft is a standard means to reconstruct defective tendons. A recent report has detailed the results of tendon allograft in reconstructing tendon defects in the hand, with a 1- to 5-year follow-up.[9] The allograft has been used when (1) patients do not want to sacrifice their own normally functioning tendons and (2) multiple tendon defects require more donor tendons than patients can offer.

The tendon has sparse cellularity and theoretically lower immunogenicity than most other tissues, and the preservation of the tendon allograft is technically possible; these factors now allow us to proceed with exploratory clinical use. In the past, several methods have been tested for the preservation of the tendon allograft for clinical use.[10–12] The author and his colleagues performed the allograft to reconstruct hand flexor or extensor tendons in 22 patients.

Indications

Indications for tendon allografts in the author's unit are as follows[8]: (1) patients have a clear and strong wish to use allogenic tendons, instead of autogenic tendons for functional reconstruction, after the surgeon has carefully explained to them the merits and potential problems of either source of grafts; (2) need for reconstruction of multiple tendons in patients, requiring multiple donor sites if autografts are used, seen in the cases of multiple tendon losses on the dorsum of the hand and wrist or secondary reconstruction of multiple lacerated flexor tendons in the palm; and (3) reconstruction of a relatively minor function, under which circumstance patients do not want to donate their own tendons. An example is a defect in a single extensor digitorum communis tendon.

Allograft Preservation, Surgical Techniques, and Postoperative Care

The allogenic tendons were harvested and transferred to deep-frozen preservation by a commercial company under strict working guidelines with the tissue bank in the Orthopedic Institute of People's Liberation Army. The fresh tendons were washed, immersed for a short time in nutritional fluid, separately sealed in sterile bags, and preserved at $-80°$. They were fully tested to exclude infectious diseases and sterilized to prevent the risk of infection of grafts. The tendons were subjected to γ-irradiation before preservation. They were thawed the day before surgery and preserved at $0°$ overnight for use. The allograft tendons were FDP or FDS tendons or digital extensor tendons.[9]

The surgical procedure is the same as the autogenic tendon grafting, and early limited-range active finger flexion is initiated to prevent adhesions of the graft, and therapy persists to 6 to 8 weeks postoperatively.

Between August 2007 and June 2011, the author and his colleagues performed tendon allografts in 22 patients (30 grafts); these patients have been regularly followed. The longest follow-up is 5 years, and no patients complain of problems associated with allogenic grafts; functional recovery of patients is, thus far, similar to that expected after conventional tendon autograft.

PEARLS, PITFALLS, AND FUTURE PERSPECTIVES

Although primary repairs of the lacerated flexor tendon are standard practice and indications for it are widely recognized, the author brings to the attention of surgeons a very small percentage of late cases in which direct repair is possible. In these well-selected cases, the return of function can sometimes be better than that achieved with

secondary repair and can be comparable with a primary repair.

This point brings up the need for careful assessment of the tensional status of the approximated tendons regarding their suitability for the direct repair. If direct repair is to be proceeded, a strong core suture repair (6 strands or more) should be used.

Tendon lengthening in the forearm helps ease the tension over the distally placed direct suture site, which can be an adjunctive to the late repair. It is true that a case presented later than 1 month after injury should be considered for secondary tendon grafting. In fact, in a small selected group of patients (fingers), direct repair is a practical option and indications for direct repair may be extended to these fingers, in some with tendon lengthening.

Although the author used a 10-strand core repair for late repair in the palm, this is the only situation in which he has used so many strands. In the digit, the author never used a core suture of more than 6 strands and considers that either a 4- or a 6-strand core suture maintains a balance between repair strength and the negative effects of sutures.[13–16] In the palm, tendons are surrounded by looser tissues, where a little bulky repair is more acceptable, and surgeons have greater flexibility to use variations of repair methods that lend greater strength to the repair.

Currently, the author's unit uses both mini-anchor and strong, reinforced suture repairs in making a tendon-bone junction. Pull-out repairs have been rare in recent years. The newer methods provide a strong junction, representing an advance over the pull-out suture. A variety of methods are available. They remain to be compared with a pull-out suture with regard to outcomes, complications, and surgical ease. Only strong and yet simple methods will survive in the future. It is certainly time to consider replacing the pull-out suture, which risks nail damage and infection and requires secondary removal of the wire.

Allograft of the tendon is a potentially feasible method for some patients who require tendon reconstruction. The author's unit set out to try this type of graft 5 years ago and has monitored this group of patients. Thus far, the author has found no significant problems with deep freeze–dried preserved allograft tendons. Nevertheless, continued lengthy follow-up is necessary to determine the long-term outcomes.

SUMMARY

The author describes a few of the uncommon methods that he has used in flexor tendon repair. Because clinical cases vary considerably, some situations may merit more unusual methods. These methods may offer alternatives to what is typically described or taught, although some should not be considered routine practice. They work well in appropriately chosen patients. The newer tendon-bone junction methods exemplified here would likely replace the pull-out suture. Late direct repair and lengthening plasty require the accumulation of clinical experience. Allograft tendon reconstruction has shown successful midterm results thus far, but long-term follow-up is certainly necessary.

REFERENCES

1. Wu YF, Tang JB. Effects of tension across the tendon repair site on tendon gap and ultimate strength. J Hand Surg Am 2012;37:906–12.

2. Tang JB, Tang JB. Indications, methods, postoperative motion and outcome evaluation of primary flexor tendon repairs in zone 2. J Hand Surg Eur 2007;32:118–29.

3. Le Viet D. Flexor tendon lengthening by tenotomy at the musculotendinous junction. Ann Plast Surg 1986;17:239–46.

4. Tripathi AK, Mee SN, Martin DL, et al. The "transverse intraosseous loop technique" (TILT) to re-insert flexor tendons in zone 1. J Hand Surg Eur 2009;34:85–9.

5. Bonin N, Obert L, Jeunet L, et al. Reinsertion of the flexor tendon using a suture anchor: prospective study using early active motion. Chir Main 2003;22:305–11 [in French].

6. Park MJ, Shin SS. Use of suture anchors and new suture materials in the upper extremity. Hand Clin 2012;28:511–8.

7. Wilson S, Sammut D. Flexor tendon graft attachment: a review of methods and a newly modified tendon graft attachment. J Hand Surg Br 2003;28:116–20.

8. Sood MK, Elliot D. A new technique of attachment of flexor tendons to the distal phalanx without a button tie-over. J Hand Surg Br 1996;21:629–32.

9. Xie RG, Tang JB. Allograft tendon for second-stage tendon reconstruction. Hand Clin 2012;28:503–9.

10. Potenza AD, Melone C. Evaluation of freeze-dried flexor tendon grafts in the dog. J Hand Surg Am 1978;3:157–62.

11. Minami A, Ishii S, Ogino T, et al. Effect of the immunological antigenicity of the allogeneic tendons on tendon grafting. Hand 1982;14:111–9.

12. Webster DA, Werner FW. Mechanical and functional properties of implanted freeze-dried flexor tendons. Clin Orthop Relat Res 1983;180:301–9.

13. Lee SK. Modern tendon repair techniques. Hand Clin 2012;28:565–70.

14. Tang JB. Clinical outcomes associated with flexor tendon repair. Hand Clin 2005;21:199–210.

15. Sandow MJ, McMahon M. Active mobilisation following single cross grasp four-strand flexor tenorrhaphy (Adelaide repair). J Hand Surg Eur 2011;36:467–75.

16. Lalonde DH. Wide-awake flexor tendon repair. Plast Reconstr Surg 2009;123:623–5.

Two-stage Reconstruction with the Modified Paneva-Holevich Technique

Kieran O'Shea, MB, FRCSI[a], Scott W. Wolfe, MD[b],*

KEYWORDS

- Flexor • Tendon • Staged • Reconstruction • Paneva-Holevich

KEY POINTS

- In the setting of flexor tendon injury, if favorable conditions for reconstruction in a single stage are not present, a staged reconstruction may be considered.
- The modified Paneva-Holevich technique, using a pedicled intra-synovial graft, is a safe and reliable means of staged flexor tendon reconstruction, offering a number of theoretical advantages over conventional free-tendon grafting techniques.
- Although no directly comparative studies exist, clinical outcomes following the Modified Paneva-Holevich Technique appear equivalent, if not superior to those achieved following classic free tendon grafting techniques.

INTRODUCTION

Flexor tendon reconstruction poses both a technical challenge to the hand surgeon and a rehabilitative challenge to the patient and therapist. When a patient presents on a delayed basis for treatment of a flexor tendon injury, or if a primary repair has failed due to either re-rupture or stiffness from adhesion formation, a single or staged reconstruction may be considered.

In proposing a severity grading system for evaluating outcome following staged flexor tendon reconstruction, Boyes[1,2] outlined the prerequisites for reconstruction in a single stage (**Table 1**). These prerequisites comprise the presence of a healed wound, supple joints with full passive mobility, absence of significant scarring in the tendon bed, and an intact flexor retinacular pulley system.

If favorable conditions for a reconstruction in a single stage are not present, then a staged reconstruction may be considered. Staged reconstruction using a tendon graft respects Bunnell's principle by placing tenorrhaphy sites outside of

zone II, where tendon adhesions are most likely to occur.[3] Beyond the second stage, a tenolysis may be required if active digital motion lags behind passive to such a degree that function is impaired. Salvage treatments, such as arthrodesis or amputation, remain reasonable options for patients who are unwilling or unable to commit to such treatment programs and their associated rehabilitation regimens.

As pioneered by Hunter and Salisbury,[4] classic staged flexor reconstruction involves the use of an extrinsic free donor tendon graft placed at the second stage following a first-stage implantation of a flexible silicone gliding implant. Potential sources for the donor intercalary graft include palmaris longus, plantaris, extensor digiti minimi, extensor indicis proprius, or the extensor digitorum longus to the second toe.[5,6] Many authors have reported reliable and satisfactory results with this technique.[7–12]

In 1965, Paneva-Holevich[13] reported her initial experience with a two-stage tenoplasty, the first stage of which involved the creation of a loop

[a] Department of Orthopaedic Surgery, St Vincents University Hospital, Elm Park, Dublin 4, Ireland;
[b] Department of Hand and Upper Extremity Surgery, Hospital for Special Surgery, Weill Cornell Medical College, 535 East 70th Street, New York, NY 10021, USA
* Corresponding author.
E-mail address: wolfes@hss.edu

Hand Clin 29 (2013) 223–233
http://dx.doi.org/10.1016/j.hcl.2013.02.011

Table 1
Boyes classification

Grade	
I	Good: minimal scar with mobile joints and no trophic changes
II	Cicatrix: heavy skin scarring from injury or previous surgery; deep scarring due to failed primary repair or infection
III	Joint damage: injury to joint with decreased range of motion
IV	Nerve damage: digital nerve injury
V	Multiple system injury; combination of above

between the proximal stumps of flexor digitorum profundus (FDP) and flexor digitorum superficialis (FDS) in the palm (**Fig. 1**A). Following a 1-month interval, a second-stage procedure was then performed consisting of division of the FDS tendon in the forearm at the musculotendinous junction. The most proximal portion of the FDS tendon was then shuttled through the pulley system and attached to the profundus stump at the distal

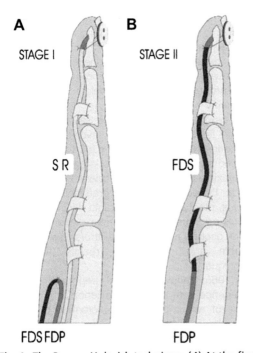

Fig. 1. The Paneva-Holevich technique. (A) At the first stage, a loop is created between the sublimis and profundus tendons in the palm. (B) At the second stage, using the profundus muscle as a motor, the sublimis tendon is routed through the pulley system, attaching to the distal phalanx. SR, silicone rod.

phalanx, acting as a pedicled intrasynovial tendon graft (see **Fig. 1**B).

Chong and colleagues[14] hypothesized that the encouraging results reported by Paneva-Holevich could be further enhanced by implanting Hunter rods at the first stage, thereby inducing the formation of a smooth sheath for tendon gliding. In 1972, both he and Kessler[15] separately found satisfactory results in small series of patients treated with this modification, which has subsequently become known as the modified Paneva-Holevich technique.

Compared with the classic 2-staged free tendon grafting, the Paneva-Holevich (PH) technique has several potential advantages, as follows:

- Intrasynovial grafts display superior morphologic and functional characteristics to conventional extrasynovial donors. They retain normal cellularity and collagen organization and heal with minimal adhesion formation, thereby providing a smooth gliding surface. Animal studies have suggested that extrasynovial grafts heal with ingrowth of peripheral adhesions that became larger and denser over time.[16–20]
- The donor FDS tendon is a better size match for the profundus tendon than the conventional extrasynovial donors, which are smaller in caliber and may be absent in up to 25% of patients.[6]
- As the FDS tendon graft is identified at the first stage, it is possible to select a silicone rod that is appropriately matched in size. In a similar manner, pulley reconstruction may be tailored to the chosen caliber of silicone implant.
- In conventional 2-stage reconstruction, difficulty is frequently encountered in identifying the profundus stump at the second stage. With the PH technique, the looped anastomosis between FDS and FDP in the palm has adequate bulk, rendering it easy to find as left at the level of the lumbricals. Relatively minor manipulation at the proximal suture line is required, further decreasing the risk for adhesions.
- Following the first-stage proximal tenorrhaphy, co-contraction of the forearm muscles simultaneously advances both tendons proximally. With relaxation, the anastomosis is returned to its resting position. By the second stage, the FDS-FDP loop has been subjected to load for 3 months on average and has completely healed. The risk of proximal rupture and failure is thereby effectively eliminated.

- Following the second stage, as only the distal tenorrhaphy has to heal, more favorable conditions for early rehabilitation are provided. As a result, a more aggressive protocol of postoperative therapy may be adopted.
- Donor site morbidity is minimized as the graft itself is truly expendable.
- Versatility is retained. Should technical difficulties be encountered at the second stage, the technique may be abandoned and the procedure converted to the classic free grafting technique.

A theoretical disadvantage of the PH technique is that it may be more difficult to judge tension at the distal anchorage point in the finger.

INDICATIONS

The principal indication for the PH technique is a chronic, neglected, Boyes grade 2 to 5, two-tendon laceration in Verdan's zone 2 with resultant nonfunctional digital flexors.[21] It may also be used for injuries in zones 3 and 4 as well as zone 1, whereby particularly in the case of the little finger, the FDS may be small or functionally absent. If a primary repair, a single- or 2-stage classic free tendon grafting procedure has failed; the PH technique may be equally used. A less frequent indication arises following digital replantation, when the fibro-osseous canal has been widely damaged or scarred. Similarly, in the acute setting, crush injuries, fractures, or infection may act as contraindications to reconstruction at or around the time of initial injury.

The ideal patient may have a scarred tendon bed but will have supple joints and good quality soft tissue cover and be strongly motivated to succeed (**Fig. 2**A, B). At the preoperative consultation, it is important to explain carefully the anticipated duration of rehabilitation and the potential for a less than perfect result.

Extensive posttraumatic palmar scarring around the expected site of the proximal anastomosis is a relative contraindication to performing the PH technique.[22] General contraindications, as per any 2-stage reconstruction, include an intact FDS tendon, a potentially poorly compliant patient, poor skin coverage (see **Fig. 2**C), and the diffuse presence of dense scar tissue. Hunter and Salisbury,[4] commenting on the merits of 2-stage reconstruction, stated, "fingers, which are stiff, as the result of severe injury or repeated unsuccessful operations, cannot be benefited by this procedure. Restoration of a tendon sheath and a gliding tendon will not mobilize a stiff finger." In this category of patients, the extent of the initial injury rather than the technique that is applied is frequently the better determinant of the final result.

SURGICAL TECHNIQUE
Stage 1

A key principle of staged reconstruction is to perform as much of the procedure as is possible at the first stage, such that the second stage requires only the passage and fixation of the tendon graft.[14]

Under regional or general anesthesia and tourniquet control, the fibro-osseous digital flexor sheath is exposed via a volar Bruner incision (**Fig. 3**).[23] Scarred portions of the flexor tendon and sheath are excised maintaining, if possible, at least 5 mm of the A2 and A4 pulleys each.[24] Next, any digital nerve injury requiring repair is addressed. Passive joint mobility is then assessed (**Fig. 4**). If a residual flexion contracture of more than 20° persists at the proximal interphalangeal joint, then an arthrolysis should be performed.[25] The volar plate is released in the first instance. If satisfactory extension is not restored following this maneuver, a capsulotomy may be considered. In the unlikely event that proximal interphalangeal joint laxity with hyperextension is encountered, a

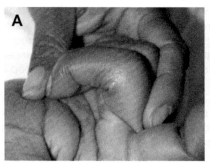
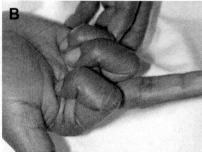
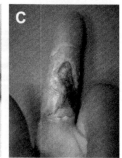

Fig. 2. (*A, B*) Ideal indication for the PH technique: supple joints with normal soft tissues. (*C*) In contrast, inadequate soft tissues are a poor indication.

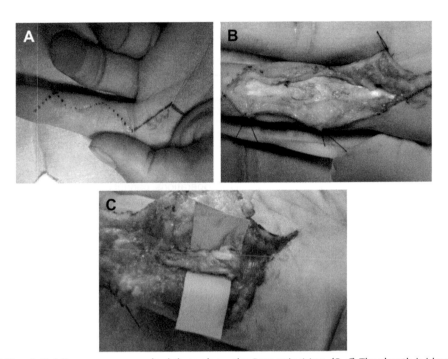

Fig. 3. (*A*) The digital flexors are approached through a volar Bruner incision. (*B, C*) The sheath is identified and scarred portions of the sheath and tendon are excised.

tenodesis may be performed on one tail of the FDS tendon may be tenodesed to the proximal to the phalanx or A2 pulley.[26]

A silicone tendon implant is then selected, approximating in size the caliber of the superficialis tendon, which will ultimately be attached to the profundus stump (**Fig. 5**A). This silicone implant acts as a passive gliding prosthesis, inducing the formation of a pseudo-sheath. A larger-sized rather than smaller-sized implant is favored so as to prevent any difficulty in shuttling the FDS tendon through the sheath at the second stage. The proximal end of the implant extends as far as the distal palmar crease and is not sutured to the lumbrical muscle.

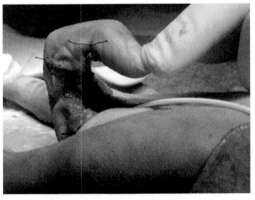

Fig. 4. Full passive digital mobility is confirmed.

Distally, the tendon implant is sutured directly to the profundus stump (see **Fig. 5**B). If there is concern in relation to the quality of fixation distally, reinforcement may be performed by means of a pullout suture placed over a button dorsally.

Attention is then directed toward the flexor retinacular pulley system. There is no clear consensus as to the extent to which pulley reconstruction should be performed. Alnot and colleagues[27] and Weinstein and colleagues[26] have stated that 4 pulleys are necessary: one proximal to each joint and one placed at the base of the proximal phalanx. Although 3 intact pulleys may be desirable, at the very least, if deficient, the A2 and A4 pulleys should be reconstructed.[4,25–27] Remnants of the excised tendons or palmaris longus may be used as grafts for pulley reconstruction. From a strength perspective, the loop or Kleinert-Weilby techniques are preferred (see **Fig. 5**C).[28–30] If a loop reconstruction is used, a triple loop is routed deep to the extensor at the proximal phalangeal level.[31] For the middle phalanx, a double loop is sufficient passing around and superficial to the extensor tendon dorsally. A caveat of this technique is that the encircling loop techniques are not suitable for use in the pediatric population. It is critical that the flexor pulley reconstructions are appropriately tensioned, because overtightening will result in stiffness due to poor gliding. If tension is insufficient, incompetence of the

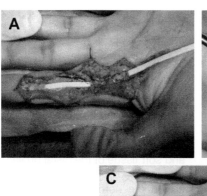
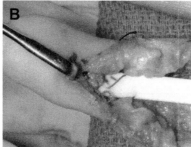
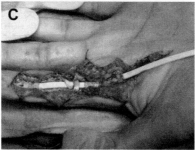

Fig. 5. (A) An appropriately sized Hunter rod is placed along the length of the flexor sheath. (B) The rod is sutured to the profundus stump distally. (C) Flexor retinacular pulley reconstruction, using the Kleinert-Weilby techique.

pulley system will lead to flexor bowstringing, loss of flexion, and predisposition to recurrent contractures.[12]

Finally, the proximal stumps of the superficialis and profundus tendons are sutured together (Fig. 6). This procedure is performed at the level of the lumbrical origin so as to ultimately avoid impingement of the proximal anastomosis against the flexor pulley system in digital extension. The tenorrhaphy site is then covered with the lumbrical muscle. The tourniquet is released. Hemostasis is confirmed and the wound is closed in the standard fashion.

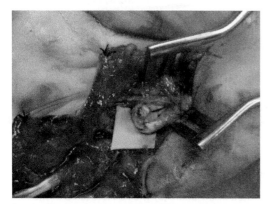

Fig. 6. The profundus and sublimis tendons are sutured together in the palm at the level of the lumbrical muscles.

After First-Stage Rehabilitation

A dorsal resting splint is applied with the wrist in 30° of flexion, the metacarpophalangeal joints in 70° flexion, and the interphalangeal joints in slightly flexed positions. Passive flexion with active extension is commenced on the third postoperative day. The aim is to achieve normal gliding of the silicone rod and full passive digital flexion and maintain this until the second-stage reconstruction. Concomitant attempts are made to address any residual flexion contractures, which, if not corrected at this stage, will have limited, if any, potential for further improvement.[32]

During this period, the patient should be closely observed for the development of flexor sheath synovitis which may result from overactivity or excessive mobility of the tendon implant, mechanical obstruction to proximal gliding, or implant buckling as a result of scarring or overtensioning of the pulley system.[33]

The cardinal features of silicone-induced synovitis include pain in the tip of the finger, swelling along the volar surface of the finger, as well as swelling and erythema in the palm. If unchecked, septic flexor tenosynovitis may supervene.[7] Initial treatment consists of rest for a period of 1 week. Failure of resolution may require an earlier than expected conversion to the second stage. Because use of an active prosthesis was associated with higher incidence of synovitis, these are no longer recommended.

Progression to the second stage can occur once maximal passive digital mobility has been achieved. A minimal interval of 3 months is preferred between stages.

Stage 2

The palmar incision is opened and the tendon anastomosis is located (see **Fig. 7**A). Any excess bulk at the site is debrided. Sheath thickening due to synovitis may be encountered and it may be necessary to release adhesions around the palmar FDS-FDP junction if they have occurred.

If, as is usual, the FDP muscle is chosen to act as the motor muscle for the finger, then the FDS is identified through a longitudinal incision in the forearm and divided at the musculotendinous junction (see **Fig. 7**B). Traction at the site of the palmar FDS-FDP anastomosis delivers the FDS tendon into the palm, where it is sutured to the

proximal end of the silicone rod (see **Fig. 7**C). An angular incision is then made at the level of the distal phalanx. It may be necessary to sacrifice the A5 pulley to achieve sufficient exposure.[24] The distal attachment of the silicone rod is identified and liberated. With traction on the rod, the FDS tendon is shuttled through the pulley system to its distal phalangeal insertion site.

The tension of the distal graft is provisionally evaluated by transfixing the tendon into the skin and soft tissue of the distal phalanx using a hypodermic needle. Tension is adjusted so as to recreate the normal cascade whereby the index finger is noted to lie in the least flexion and the little finger is noted to lie in the most flexion. It is advisable to position the digit in a slightly greater degree of flexion, as opposed to lesser degree, so as to allow for creep, and the resultant small amount of lengthening that may occur with time. The ability to achieve full passive digital extension is verified.

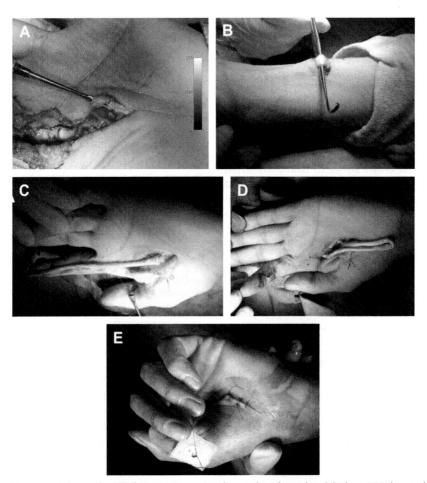

Fig. 7. (*A*) At the second stage, the tendon anastomosis is located in the palm. (*B*) The FDS is located in the forearm and divided at the musculotendinous junction. (*C*) Traction at the anastomosis delivers the FDS tendon into the palm. (*D*) The FDS has been shuttled through the flexor retinacular pulley system (*E*) Distal attachment of the FDS using sutures tied over a dorsal button at the distal phalanx.

Observing the tenodesis effect is useful as a further means to evaluate the appropriateness of graft tensioning.

A variety of options exist for the fixation of the distal tendon insertion site. If a 1-cm stump of the FDP has been retained, a simple end-to-end repair may be performed. Although contraindicated in skeletally immature patients, another option is to create a bony tunnel insertion site at the distal phalanx. Our preference is to secure the tendon in a manner similar to that used during repair of an FDP avulsion, by passing a 3-0 Prolene suture from the tendon from volar to dorsal through the bone of the distal phalanx and tying over a dorsal button (see **Fig. 7**D). To minimize the potential for nail deformities, the needle and suture are passed proximal to the germinal matrix of the distal phalanx. The stump of the FDP may then be incorporated into the FDS tendon, reinforcing the repair volarly.

After Second-Stage Rehabilitation

A resting splint is applied in a similar manner to that following the first-stage reconstruction. An early controlled motion rehabilitation protocol is commenced incorporating passive flexion and active extension and maintaining joint mobility. Active flexion is commenced at 4 weeks and the dorsal button is removed at 6 weeks, after which time unprotected digital motion is allowed. Full, unrestricted use including flexion against resistance is delayed until 4 months postoperatively.

Closely supervised hand therapy is integral to ensuring a positive outcome following staged flexor tendon reconstruction. Naam[32] reported inferior results in those patients who were noncompliant or could not readily access therapy for geographic reasons. If, after a minimum interval period of 3 months, satisfactory active motion has not been restored, a third-stage procedure consisting of a tenolysis may be considered (**Fig. 8**). It should be noted that the results of tenolysis are unpredictable. A single-level improvement, using the outcome measures proposed by Strickland and Buck-Gramco, will typically occur in 50% of patients.[34–36] Amadio and colleagues[7] reported an average net improvement in flexion of 22° in their cohort following tenolysis.

MODIFICATIONS

The PH technique may be adapted for staged superficialis finger reconstruction, whereby the tendon graft is anchored distally to the middle phalanx.[37] In the primary setting, a superficialis reconstruction may be considered if there is poor quality soft tissue cover overlying the distal phalanx or in the presence of severe stiffness or destruction of the distal interphalangeal joint. Superficialis reconstruction may also be used as a salvage procedure following graft failure at the distal phalangeal insertion site.

It may arise that the donor FDS tendon of the digit to be reconstructed is deficient or, as in the case of the little finger, absent in approximately 9% of cases.[38] In this setting, an FDS graft may be harvested from an adjacent injured or noninjured digit. If a poor-quality graft is encountered, an alternative option is to harvest a palmaris longus graft for use as reinforcement.

Finally, in the setting of staged thumb flexor tendon reconstruction following zone II injuries, a modified PH technique may be performed whereby a loop is created between the flexor pollicis longus and palmaris longus in the distal forearm at the first stage.[39]

COMPLICATIONS

Complications are common following staged flexor tendon reconstruction, with a 41% incidence reported by Wehbe and colleagues.[12]

Although failure occurs more commonly at the distal attachment than proximally, one of the principal advantages of the PH technique is that the risk of re-rupture at the proximal anastomotic site is virtually eliminated.[21,32] With conventional 2-stage reconstruction using a free tendon graft, the incidence of rupture has been reported at between 4% and 14%.[6,12,25,40] If proximal rupture occurs, an end-to-side repair to a neighboring tendon in the palm may be performed. In the case of distal rupture, revision to a middle phalangeal insertion site, creating a superficialis finger, is preferred, although re-grafting with a palmaris longus tendon graft is an alternative option.

As alluded to previously, one potential disadvantage of the PH technique is that it may be more difficult to judge and set tension at the distal anastomosis. The tendency is toward undertensioning rather than overtensioning. If it is evident, during the postoperative period, that a slack graft has been placed, it is possible to re-tension by performing a tendon-shortening procedure proximal to the wrist.

Postoperative persistent flexion contractures, ranging in magnitude from 8° to 55°, were reported by Naam and colleagues[32] in 88% of cases following reconstruction using the modified PH technique. The presence of a preoperative contracture is the most predictive feature in determining the presence of a postoperative contracture. Incompetency of the flexor retinacular pulley system is a further contributing or compounding

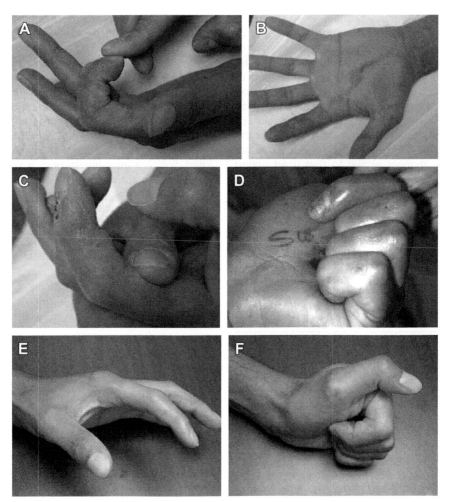

Fig. 8. (*A–C*) Although full passive digital motion is possible, significant restriction in active flexion persists at 3 months post staged flexor reconstruction. (*D*) Post tenolysis, near full active flexion is possible. (*E, F*) At 16 weeks, although mild flexion contractures remain, near complete digital flexion is maintained.

factor.[25] Closely supervised hand therapy and the use of pulley rings, when the condition and swelling of the soft tissues permit, may be helpful in minimizing this problem.

Historically, distal interphalangeal joint contractures were observed primarily following dynamic traction splinting rehabilitation protocols.[32,41] It is thought that current early controlled active motion protocols may reduce their incidence and severity. Distal interphalangeal joint arthrodesis may be considered for recalcitrant contractures.

Infection has a reported incidence of between 5% and 15% but is clearly associated with poorer clinical outcome and carries with it a risk of amputation.[7,12,42] If arising during the first stage and detected early, it may respond to intravenous antibiotic administration and closed irrigation drainage of the pseudo-sheath.[21,25] If well established, formal debridement with removal of the silicone rod is needed. A repeat first-stage reconstruction

may later be performed, following a minimum 6-month interval, to be confident that sepsis has been eradicated.

DISCUSSION

In their 1983 report from the Committee on Tendon Injuries, Kleinert and Verdan[36] acknowledged the role held by the PH technique in staged flexor tendon reconstruction. The widespread adoption of the classic Hunter technique seems to have limited its incorporation into many hand surgeons' practices.

Although no studies have been performed directly comparing the 2 techniques, the results following the PH technique seem equivalent if not superior to those reported with classic staged free tendon grafting. Difficulties in comparison are compounded by the lack of consistency in the outcome measures that have been used for

Table 2
Paneva-Holevich technique: Results in the literature to date

Study	n (Digits) in Zone II	Evaluation	Good and Excellent Results (%)
Kessler,[15] 1972	6	Strickland[a]	83
Winspur et al,[43] 1978	10	Buck-Gramcko[a]	80
Brug et al,[44] 1979	27	Buck-Gramcko	52
Chuinard et al,[37] 1980 (superficialis finger)	16	Boyes (modified)	62.5
Paneva-Holevich,[45] 1982	39	Boyes (modified)	56[a]
Alnot et al,[27] 1996	19	Total active motion–total active extension deficit	73[a]
Naam,[32] 1997	21	Strickland and Glogovac	52.4
Brug et al,[46] 1998	76	Buck-Gramcko	55
Beris et al,[21] 2003	22	Buck-Gramcko	82
		Modified Strickland	73

[a] Calculated based on data provided in the original articles.
Data from Beris AE, Darlis NA, Korompilias AV, et al. Two-stage flexor tendon reconstruction in zone II using a silicone rod and a pedicled intrasynovial graft. J Hand Surg Am 2003;28:652–60.

evaluation. In addition, the wide spectrum of severity of these injuries cannot be readily controlled for and postoperative therapy has varied from earlier immobilization-based to more recent controlled active motion regimes.

In a series of 117 two-stage digital flexor reconstructions using a classic free tendon graft, Amadio and colleagues[7] reported 54% good to excellent results using the LaSalle and Strickland scale. The percentage of zone 2 injuries experiencing good to excellent results was 42%. Nineteen percent of digits had a total active motion (TAM) of greater than 180°. Tenolysis was performed in 16% of cases with a net average improvement in TAM active motion from pretenolysis to posttenolysis of 22°. Graft rupture was observed in 4%.

LaSalle and Strickland[42] reported a series of 43 patients, with good to excellent results observed in 39% of cases. Forty-seven percent of patients required a third-stage tenolysis. Evaluating the posttenolysis results improved the overall outcome such that 65% were rated good to excellent.

Weinstein and colleagues,[26] in evaluating 32 digits, reported 60.9% good, 21.7% fair, and 17.4% poor results in terms of the total active flexion achieved. Wehbe and colleagues,[12] reporting on 150 patients, found that the average TAM improved from 102° to 176°. Tenolysis was required in 12% and tendon rupture occurred in 14%.

In comparison, **Table 2** outlines the results following the PH technique as reported in the literature to date.[14,21,26,32,37,43–46] Although the lack of consistency in study methodology has been previously acknowledged, good to excellent results were reported in between 73% and 82% of cases when the Strickland scale was used.

Using the modified PH technique, Beris and colleagues[21] reported a mean achieved total active digital range of motion of 189°, equivalent to 71% that of the contralateral respective finger. Distal graft rupture occurred in 1 of 22 patients. There was no instance of proximal rupture and no patient required a third-stage tenolysis.

Naam[32] reported an improvement of greater than 50% in digital active range of motion in 64% of patients. Although 3 of 47 patients required tenolysis, there was no incidence of proximal or distal graft rupture.

SUMMARY

The modified PH technique, using a pedicled intrasynovial graft, is a safe and reliable means of staged flexor tendon reconstruction. It offers several theoretical advantages over the classic free-tendon grafting techniques. Donor morbidity is minimized as the graft itself is expendable. The donor FDS more closely matches the size of the injured profundus tendon and the FDS tendon can be identified at the first stage, facilitating selection of appropriately sized Hunter rods and the appropriate tensioning of pulley reconstructions. As the proximal anastomosis is healed by the second stage, the risk of rupture at this site is effectively eliminated. Clinical outcomes are at the least comparable, if not superior, with this technique and most authors report a low requirement for third-stage tenolysis.

REFERENCES

1. Boyes JH. Flexor tendon grafts in the fingers and thumb: an evaluation of end results. J Bone Joint Surg Am 1950;32:489–99.

2. Boyes JH, Stark HH. Flexor tendon grafts in the fingers and thumb: a study of factors influencing results in 1000 cases. J Bone Joint Surg Am 1971; 53:1332–42.

3. Bunnell S. Bunnell's surgery of the hand. Revised by JH Boyes. 4th edition. Philadelphia: J. B. Lippincott; 1964.

4. Hunter JM, Salisbury RE. Flexor tendon reconstruction in severely damaged hands: a two-stage procedure using a silicone-Dacron reinforced gliding prosthesis prior to tendon grafting. J Bone Joint Surg Am 1971;53:829–58.

5. Wehbé MA. Tendon graft anatomy and harvesting. Orthop Rev 1994;23:253–6.

6. Carlson GD, Botte MJ, Josephs MS, et al. Morphologic and biomechanical comparison of tendons used as free grafts. J Hand Surg Am 1993;18:76–82.

7. Amadio PC, Wood MB, Cooney WP III, et al. Staged flexor tendon reconstruction in the fingers and hand. J Hand Surg Am 1988;13:559–62.

8. Chamay A, Verdan C, Simonetta C. Les greffes de tendons flechisseurs après implantation provisoire d'une tige en silicone. Etude et resultats de 32 cas. Rev Chir Orthop Reparatrice Appar Mot 1975;61:599–610 [in French].

9. Honner R, Meares A. A review of 100 flexor tendon reconstructions with prosthesis. Hand 1977;9:226–31.

10. Hunter JM. Staged flexor tendon reconstruction. J Hand Surg Am 1983;8:789–93.

11. Valenti P, Gilbert A. Two-stage flexor tendon grafting in children. Hand Clin 2000;16:573–8.

12. Wehbe MA, Hunter JM, Schneider LH, et al. Two-stage flexor-tendon reconstruction: ten-year experience. J Bone Joint Surg Am 1986;68:752–63.

13. Paneva-Holevich E. Two-stage plasty in flexor tendon injuries of fingers within the digital synovial sheath. Acta Chir Plast 1965;7:112–24.

14. Chong JK, Cramer LM, Culf NK. Combined two-stage tenoplasty with silicone rods for multiple flexor tendon injuries in "no-man's land." J Trauma 1972; 12:104–21.

15. Kessler FB. Use of a pedicled tendon transfer with a silicone rod in complicated secondary flexor tendon repairs. Plast Reconstr Surg 1972;49:439–43.

16. Lundborg G. Experimental flexor tendon healing without adhesion formation: a new concept of tendon nutrition and intrinsic healing mechanisms. A preliminary report. Hand 1976;8:235–8.

17. Abrahamsson SO, Gelberman RH, Lohmander SL. Variations in cellular proliferation and matrix synthesis in intrasynovial and extrasynovial tendons: an in vitro study in dogs. J Hand Surg Am 1994;19:259–65.

18. Gelberman RH, Seiler JG III, Rosenberg AE, et al. Intercalary flexor tendon grafts: a morphological study of intrasynovial and extrasynovial donor tendons. Scand J Plast Reconstr Surg Hand Surg 1992;26:257–64.

19. Seiler JG III, Gelberman RH, Williams CS, et al. Autogenous flexor tendon grafts: a biomechanical and morphological study in dogs. J Bone Joint Surg Am 1993;75:1004–14.

20. Seiler JG III, Chu CR, Amiel D, et al. Autogenous flexor tendon grafts. Biologic mechanisms for incorporation. Clin Orthop Relat Res 1997;345:239–47.

21. Beris AE, Darlis NA, Korompilias AV, et al. Two-stage flexor tendon reconstruction in zone II using a silicone rod and a pedicled intrasynovial graft. J Hand Surg Am 2003;28:652–60.

22. Paneva-Holevich E. Two-stage tenoplasty in injury of the flexor tendons of the hand. J Bone Joint Surg Am 1969;51:21–32.

23. Bruner JM. The zig-zag volar-digital incision for flexor tendon surgery. Plast Reconstr Surg 1967; 40:571–4.

24. Goldfarb CA, Gelberman RH, Boyer MI. Flexor tendon reconstruction: current concepts and techniques. J Hand Surg Am 2005;5:123–30.

25. Schneider LH. Staged flexor tendon reconstruction using the method of Hunter. Clin Orthop Relat Res 1982;171:164–71.

26. Weinstein SL, Sprague BL, Flatt AE. Evaluation of the two-stage flexor-tendon reconstruction in severely damaged digits. J Bone Joint Surg Am 1976;58: 786–91.

27. Alnot JY, Mouton P, Bisson P. Longstanding flexor tendon lesions treated by two-stage tendon graft. Ann Chir Main 1996;15:25–35.

28. Hume EL, Hutchinson DL, Jeager SA, et al. Biomechanics of pulley reconstruction. J Hand Surg Am 1991;16:722–30.

29. Widstrom C, Johnson G, Doyle J, et al. A mechanical study of six pulley reconstruction techniques: part I Mechanical effectiveness. J Hand Surg Am 1989; 14:821–5.

30. Kleinert HE, Bennett JB. Digital pulley reconstruction employing the always present rim of the previous pulley. J Hand Surg Am 1978;3:297–8.

31. Okutsu I, Ninomiya S, Hiraki S, et al. Three-loop technique for A2 pulley reconstruction. J Hand Surg Am 1987;12:790–4.

32. Naam NH. Staged flexor tendon reconstruction using pedicled tendon graft from the flexor digitorum superficialis. J Hand Surg Am 1997;22:323–7.

33. Soucacos PN, Beris AE, Malizos KN, et al. Two-stage treatment of flexor tendon ruptures. Silicone

rod complications analyzed in 109 digits. Acta Orthop Scand 1997;68:48–51.

34. Strickland J. Flexor tendon surgery. Part 2: free tendon grafts and tenolysis. J Hand Surg Br 1989; 14:368–82.

35. Strickland J. Flexor tenolysis. Hand Clin 1985;1: 121–32.

36. Kleinert HE, Verdan C. Report of the committee on tendon injuries. J Hand Surg Am 1983;5:794–8.

37. Chuinard RG, Dabezies EJ, Mathews RE. Two-stage superficialis tendon reconstruction in severely damaged fingers. J Hand Surg Am 1980;5:135–43.

38. Thompson NW, Mockford BJ, Rasheed T, et al. Functional absence of flexor digitorum superficialis to the little finger and absence of palmaris longus– is there a link? J Hand Surg Br 2002;27:433–4.

39. Foucher G, Merle M, Sibilly A, et al. Flexor tendon grafting. The use of a modified Hunter's technique. Rev Chir Orthop Reparatrice Appar Mot 1978;64: 703–5 [in French].

40. Coyle MP Jr, Leddy TP, Leddy JP. Staged flexor tendon reconstruction fingertip to palm. J Hand Surg Am 2002;27:581–5.

41. Tonkin M, Hagberg L, Lister G. Post operative management of flexor tendon grafting. J Hand Surg Br 1988;13:277–81.

42. LaSalle WB, Strickland JW. An evaluation of the two-stage flexor tendon reconstruction technique. J Hand Surg Am 1983;8:263–7.

43. Winspur I, Dennis PB, Boswick JA. Staged reconstruction of flexor tendons with a silicone rod and a "pedicled" sublimis transfer. Plast Reconstr Surg 1978;61:756–61.

44. Brug E, Stedtfeld HW. Experience with a two-stage pedicled flexor tendon graft. Hand 1979;11:198–205.

45. Paneva-Holevich E. Two-stage reconstruction of the flexor tendons. Int Orthop 1982;6:133–8.

46. Brug E, Wetterkamp D, Neuber M, et al. Secondary reconstruction of flexor tendon function in the fingers. Unfallchirurg 1998;101:415–25.

Flexor Pulley Reconstruction

Christopher J. Dy, MD, MSPH, Aaron Daluiski, MD*

KEYWORDS

- Flexor pulley reconstruction • Biomechanics • Flexor tendon bowstringing

KEY POINTS

- A2 and A4 are the most important flexor pulleys to avoid flexor tendon bowstringing and are therefore the most commonly reconstructed.
- However, recent studies indicate that both A2 and A4 may not need to be fully intact to avoid bowstringing. The surgeon should be prepared to reconstruct the number of pulleys needed to maintain the flexor tendons close to the axis of motion.
- Although looped reconstruction is biomechanically stronger than reconstructions that incorporate the remnant pulley rim, the mechanical strength required for postoperative rehabilitation and normal human hand use is not known.
- It is imperative to ensure that enough tension is present in the reconstructed pulley to maintain the tendon close to the axis of motion, but not too tight to prevent tendon gliding.

OVERVIEW

The intricate anatomy and complex function of the flexor pulley system are distinctly challenging to restore after injury. A complete understanding of the normal anatomy and function is helpful in guiding treatment of flexor pulley injuries.

Flexor pulley injuries requiring surgical management are relatively uncommon. The authors' preliminary analysis of a statewide administrative database showed an average of 46 pulley reconstructions performed per year by 126 surgeons in New York State from 1997 to 2006. Based on these data, one surgeon performs a pulley reconstruction less than once every 2 years (0.4 pulley reconstructions per year per surgeon). Despite the infrequency of these injuries, surgeons need to be prepared to perform flexor pulley reconstructions because of the disability that ensues from a failed flexor pulley system.

ANATOMY

The flexor pulley system comprises the palmar aponeurosis pulley, 5 annular pulleys, and 3 cruciate pulleys. Although pulley reconstruction has been described as early as 1933,[1] Doyle and Blythe's seminal work in 1975 has informed much of the knowledge of the flexor pulley anatomy and function.[2] Their initial description of 4 annular and 3 cruciate pulleys was later revised by Hunter and colleagues,[3] who described a fifth annular pulley arising from the volar plate of the distal interphalangeal joint. Manske and Lesker subsequently described the palmar aponeurosis pulley, in which the transverse fibers of the palmar aponeurosis form an archway over the flexor tendons.[4]

The pulleys are fibrous bands with either a ring-shaped configuration, as seen in the annular pulleys, or a cruciform configuration, as seen in the cruciate pulleys. The A1, A3, and A5 pulleys originate from the volar plate and adjacent bony surfaces of the metacarpophalangeal (MCP) joint, proximal interphalangeal (PIP) joint, and the distal interphalangeal (DIP) joint, respectively. The A2 and A4 pulleys originate from, and insert onto, the bony surfaces of the proximal and middle phalanges, respectively. Although the leading edge of A2 is relatively prominent as it overlies the base of the proximal phalanx,[5] the thickest portion of A2

Division of Hand and Upper Extremity Surgery, Department of Orthopaedic Surgery, Hospital for Special Surgery, New York, NY 10021, USA
* Corresponding author. 523 East 72nd Street, New York, NY 10021.
E-mail address: daluiskia@hss.edu

Hand Clin 29 (2013) 235–242
http://dx.doi.org/10.1016/j.hcl.2013.02.005
0749-0712/13/$ – see front matter © 2013 Elsevier Inc. All rights reserved.

hand.theclinics.com

(up to 0.75 mm) is its distal end.[2] The A2 and A4 pulleys span the diaphyseal region of the proximal and middle phalanges, respectively. They are stiffer, broader, and shorten less during finger flexion than the other pulleys,[6] reflecting their function in keeping the flexor tendons close to the axis of joint motion. The average lengths of the annular pulleys are 7.9 mm (A1), 16.8 mm (A2), 2.8 mm (A3), 6.7 mm (A4), and 4.1 mm (A5).[5] These dimensions should be kept in mind when attempting to replicate the normal anatomy while reconstructing the flexor pulleys.

The cruciate pulleys are located at the distal end of A2 (C1), between A3 and A4 (C2), and at the distal end of A4 (C3). The cruciate pulleys are composed of oblique fibers that interdigitate with the adjacent annular pulleys. They are relatively flexible, allowing them to shorten or collapse during finger flexion to protect the annular pulleys.

The pulleys are composed of 3 layers, each with a distinct function[7]: the inner-most layer promotes tendon gliding by secreting hyaluronic acid; the collagen-rich middle layer provides structural support; and the outer layer provides nutrition. The complexity of the anatomy of the flexor pulley system provides insight into the challenge of restoring the normal function of the system.

FUNCTION AND BIOMECHANICS

The flexor pulley system is to maintain the flexor tendons close to the axis of motion, allowing the conversion of tendon excursion into angular motion of the joints of the fingers. There is a size discrepancy between the external diameter of the flexor tendon sheath and the internal diameter of the flexor pulley, indicating the importance of a properly tensioned and smoothly gliding interface between tendon and pulley to allow tendon excursion.

The annular pulleys minimize the amount of tendon excursion needed to provide finger flexion. If the flexor tendons fall away (bowstringing) from the phalanges because of pulley injury, the amount of distal flexion generated is compromised because the resultant tendon excursion cannot compensate for the increase in the moment arm (from the phalanx to the displaced tendon).[8]

Based on anatomic observations and biomechanical studies, most investigators agree that both A2 and A4 are most important to optimal efficiency of the flexor tendons.[5,9,10] In view of these findings, many hand surgeons consider the A2 and A4 pulleys to be inviolable and use alternate intervals between and within the other pulleys to perform flexor tendon repair. However, situations may arise in which partial or complete release of the A2 or A4 pulley is necessary to place core tendon sutures or to allow gliding of a repaired tendon.[11]

Although any compromise of A2 or A4 raises the theoretical concern for bowstringing, recent studies have suggested that A2 and A4 can be partially incised without substantial effects on work of flexion or tendon excursion.[12-15] In a cadaveric model, Mitsionis and coworkers[14] demonstrated that 25% of both A2 and A4 can be released, either alone or in conjunction, without a significant loss of finger flexion. In addition, they suggested that more aggressive release (up to 75%) may still provide finger motion that is clinically acceptable. In animal models, Tang and colleagues[16,17] have demonstrated that complete incision of the A2 pulley improved tendon excursion and decreased the work of flexion compared with intact or repaired A2 pulleys. Furthermore, Franko and colleagues[18] have shown that complete release of A4 does not substantially increase work of flexion or tendon excursion in a cadaveric model. These biomechanical studies have been supported by clinical reports advocating the intentional release of A4 to facilitate flexor tendon repair.[11,17]

These advances have provided important knowledge to surgeons faced with difficult choices during acute flexor tendon repair, but also afford insight into the relative infrequency of flexor pulley reconstruction. Although prior belief was that complete integrity of both A2 and A4 was needed for a fully functioning flexor apparatus, there seems to be a certain amount of physiologic leniency within the flexor pulley system that was not previously appreciated. Patients may be able to tolerate some compromise of their pulley system, even within A2 and A4, allowing them to avoid pulley reconstruction. Although this evolving knowledge does not change the current general indications for flexor pulley reconstruction, it allows the surgeon to tailor his or her approach, especially in regard to the number of pulleys to reconstruct.

GENERAL CONSIDERATIONS FOR RECONSTRUCTION
Clinical Presentation and Imaging

Spontaneous pulley injuries may occur after activities that involve a rapidly applied extension force to an acutely flexed digit,[19] such as rock climbing,[20,21] pitching,[22] or suddenly lifting or pulling against a heavy object.[23] Athletically active patients may present with prodromal pain and swelling along the volar aspect of the proximal phalanx in the 2 to 3 weeks before acute rupture.[24]

After the acute rupture, patients may recall something "tearing" in their finger and subsequently report pain with gripping, local tenderness, and decreased finger dexterity. Alternatively, symptoms may be limited to those associated with a developing PIP flexion contracture in the subacute time period.[19] Flexor pulley injuries may also occur in the setting of a traumatic laceration or may present after prior surgery, such as flexor tendon repair, tenolysis, or aggressive trigger finger release.[8,25] Magnetic resonance imaging[26–28] and dynamic ultrasound[29] can be useful in confirming the diagnosis of pulley rupture by visualizing displacement of the flexor tendons away from the volar surface of the phalanges (**Fig. 1**). These studies can also be helpful in excluding concurrent injuries to the flexor tendons and planning for surgical reconstruction.

Indications

Nonoperative management using a ring splint to minimize bowstringing can be successful for patients with closed single pulley ruptures (**Fig. 2**). Moutet and coworkers[24] reported success and return to baseline activities in 11 of 12 patients treated with a ring splint for 45 days. Anecdotal evidence from Bollen indicates that rock climbers with a history of pulley rupture treated with either splinting or neglect are still able to function at a competitive level, even with clinically apparent bowstringing.[30]

Surgical treatment is reserved for patients with multiple closed pulley ruptures, persistent pain, or dysfunction after attempted nonoperative management of a single pulley rupture, or during concurrent or staged flexor tendon repair or reconstruction.

Principles

If the local tissue is suitable, flexor pulley repair is desired over other options if it can be achieved without decreasing the volume available for

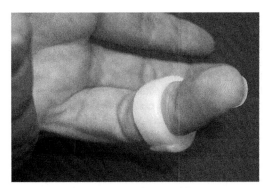

Fig. 2. Thermoplastic ring splint used for nonoperative management or postsurgical splinting. (*Courtesy of Aviva Wolff and HSS Hand Therapy, with permission.*)

tendon gliding.[31] Alternative approaches include pulley dilation, resection of a single slip of flexor digitorum superficialis (FDS),[17] V-Y plasty of the pulley,[32] and pulley enlargement with or without tendon graft.[16,33,34] The latter may be more appropriate after surgical pulley release during flexor tendon repair given that the tissue will be more amenable to graft incorporation than nonsurgically traumatized remnant pulley. Once the decision has been made to perform flexor pulley reconstruction, the surgeon must be mindful of several principles.

The intact pulley length should be replicated to maximize efficiency of the reconstructed flexor pulley.[35,36] The average lengths of A2 and A4 are 16.8 mm and 6.7 mm, respectively.[5] Approximately 6 to 8 cm of graft is needed for each pass around the phalanx[37] if a loop-around-bone technique is used. Each loop around bone provides approximately 5 mm of length. Correspondingly, 18 to 24 cm of tendon graft is needed for A2 and 12 to 16 cm of tendon graft is needed for A4.

The size mismatch between the diameter of the flexor tendon and the internal diameter of the intact pulley reflects the challenges of reconstructing the flexor system. Biomechanical studies have shown that synovial-lined grafts, such as a segment of extensor retinaculum,[38] sheath of first

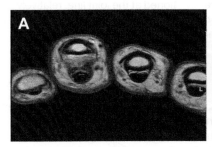
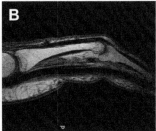

Fig. 1. Axial (*A*) and sagittal (*B*) magnetic resonance imaging images from a patient with traumatic A2 flexor pulley disruption. Note the displacement of the flexor tendons away from the volar surface of the proximal phalanx. Copyright Aaron Daluiski, MD; with permission.

dorsal compartment,[39] or a slip of FDS,[40] are superior to extrasynovial grafts in re-establishing the gliding mechanism in biomechanical studies.[41,42] Standard extrasynovial autograft options include palmaris longus and extensor tendon. Naidu and Rinkus[43] reported the use of gracilis allograft for pulley reconstruction based on patient preference over autograft. The use of synthetic grafts for pulley reconstruction was described in 1968 by Bader and colleagues,[44] who used silicone, and in 1974 by Wray and Weeks,[45] who used Dacron. The recently developed synthetic graft is polytetrafluoroethylene, which has shown favorable mechanical strength without causing adverse effects on tendon healing, adhesions, or host reaction.[46–48] All these have not been routinely used clinically. Autograft is generally preferable and available. Other options, such as bovine pericardial graft and acellular dermal matrix, have shown promising results in animal studies and may deserve future consideration.[49]

Achieving the appropriate tension within the flexor pulley is one of the most challenging aspects of performing pulley reconstruction. An ideal pulley reconstruction maintains the flexor tendons close enough to volar surface of the phalanges, but also leaves enough room for the tendon to glide freely. Brand and colleagues[50] thought that one way to assess pulley tension was to ensure that tendon excursion is equal between full extension to 30° flexion and between 60° to 90° flexion. Other authors have advised additional methods to check pulley tension, such as ensuring that a Kirschner wire can fit alongside the tendon underneath the pulley,[36] placing hemostats on the corners of a reconstructed pulley to evenly tension the pulley over the tendon,[36] or performing "wide-awake" surgery under local anesthetics to ensure tendon gliding while the patient actively flexes the finger.[8,51]

The recent advances in knowledge regarding partial release of A2 and A4 reflect the importance of customizing the number and type of pulleys to be reconstructed. The surgeon should be prepared to reconstruct the appropriate number of pulleys to ensure that the tendon glides smoothly without any evident bowstringing.

RECONSTRUCTION TECHNIQUES

There are 2 general categories of pulley reconstruction: those that do not encircle the phalanx and those that loop around the phalanx. Regarding the former, Klinert and Bennett described a technique to reconstruct the flexor pulleys using a graft woven between the "always present rim of the previous pulley."[52] This technique, which was attributed to Andreas Weilby, is often described as a "shoelace" or "interweave" reconstruction. After using a no. 11 blade to create eyelet perforations in the tissue on both remnant rims, a tendon graft is passed back and forth over the flexor tendon or silicone rod (in cases of delayed tendon reconstruction) through the eyelet perforations, much like a Pulvertaft weave (**Fig. 3**). Modern modifications include the use of a slip of flexor digitorum superficialis with a maintained distal attachment,[40] suturing extensor retinaculum graft into the remnant pulley rims without a shoelace weave,[24] and fixing a graft of extensor retinaculum with periosteum to the fibro osseous floor of the flexor sheath.[53] Tension is checked after the final weave is complete. It may be helpful to flex the finger to bring the tendons closer to the volar aspect of the phalanges before securing final tension.[24] Cadaveric experiments have shown the original Weilby technique to be mechanically weaker, with lower energy absorption and lower breaking strength, than looped repairs.[6,54] In view of Widstrom's observation that mechanical failures of the Weilby technique occurred after the tendon graft pulled out of the remnant rim,[54] the surgeon should consider both the quality and the quantity of the local tissue when deciding whether to use this technique.

Karev and coworkers[55] have described a reconstruction that can be readily used in the setting of a concurrent flexor tendon repair or staged graft/implant reconstruction. In the "belt-loop" reconstruction, 2 transverse incisions 3 to 5 mm apart are made in the volar plate of the metacarpalphalangeal, PIP, or DIP joints. The authors have emphasized the importance of palpating the softness and elasticity of the volar plate before using this technique to check its suitability as a pulley.[56] Before tenorrhaphy, the tendon is passed underneath the roof created by the communication between the transverse incisions. The repaired tendon is prevented from bowstringing by the overlying belt-loop roof. Because the roof is positioned at the joint line, relatively little tendon excursion is required. Although successful at preventing

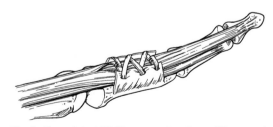

Fig. 3. Completed Weilby reconstruction of flexor pulley. Copyright Aaron Daluiski, MD; with permission.

bowstringing[55] and stronger than the Weilby shoelace reconstruction, it is not as strong as looped reconstructions.[54] In addition, the volar plate forms a relatively stiff roof, creating substantial increases in friction and work of flexion during tendon gliding. The long-term effects of the reconstruction on the volar plate and corresponding articulation have not been described, but loss of volar plate function and articular erosion have been reported.[57] Although it has its limitations, the Karev belt-loop reconstruction may have its particular advantages when the need arises to reconstruct the A1, A3, or A5 pulleys in the setting of staged tendon grafting.

The other major category of flexor pulley reconstruction involves passing a loop of graft around the phalanx (**Fig. 4**). Although the first published description of using a looped tendon graft to reconstruct the flexor pulley is attributed to Bunnell,[58] many prefer the modification described by Okutsu and colleagues[35] that uses 3 separate loops around the proximal phalanx. The additional loops are intended to increase pulley length, and this has been confirmed in cadaveric studies comparing the 3-loop reconstruction to single-loop, belt-loop, and Weilby techniques.[6,54]

After a volar approach to the tendon, a tenolysis is performed with particular care taken to excise any scar or adhesion behind the tendon. The lateral borders of the phalanx are exposed, taking care to retract the adjacent neurovascular structures. When reconstructing A2, the graft is passed between the extensor mechanism and the dorsal aspect of the proximal phalanx. However, when reconstructing A4, the graft is passed around the entirety of the extensor mechanism. A right-angled clamp or curved suture passer can be used to facilitate passage of the tendon graft. The position of the pulley reconstruction and the number of loop passes are based on the location and length of the native pulley. After each pass of the graft, the surgeon has the opportunity to check and adjust the tension of the pulley reconstruction. Passively flexing the finger before suturing each loop may be helpful to keep the flexor tendons as close to bone as possible during adjustment of pulley tension.[24] It is imperative to ensure enough tension to maintain the tendon close to the axis of motion, but not too tight to

prevent tendon gliding. Passive finger flexion is checked and active motion is evaluated if the patient is awake during surgery. After tension is deemed to be adequate, the reconstructed pulley loops are sutured to themselves and to the remaining local tissue.

For A4 reconstructions, passing the graft superficial to the extensor tendons may compromise motion of the extensor mechanism. For A2 reconstructions, passing the graft directly along the proximal phalanx raises the theoretical concern of vascular compromise to the flexor tendons[35] and potential bone resorption underneath the pulley graft.[59] The addition of more loops to the pulley reconstruction helps to match the native pulley length and strength.[6] Surgeons must balance the demand for pulley strength with these potential risks. Although 2 loops may provide enough strength to allow early motion, this may not give enough length to match the native pulley length, especially for A2. The superior biomechanical properties of the triple-loop reconstruction have prompted some surgeons to use this technique because of its immediate strength.[6,8,37] However, the mechanical strength of a pulley required for postoperative active tendon motion and normal hand use is not known.

Other looped reconstruction techniques include Lister's single loop of extensor retinaculum and Widstrom's loop-and-a-half technique. The former provides a smooth gliding surface[41] but is limited by its inferior biomechanical strength compared with looped reconstruction.[54] In the loop-and-a-half technique, one limb of the graft is passed around the phalanx and passed through the other limb of the graft. Although has equivalent biomechanical effectiveness to single-loop reconstructions, it has not been widely used because of concerns for its inability to prevent bowstringing.[54]

Recently a hybrid approach was developed to pulley reconstruction with a half-loop of graft secured to bone with suture anchors.[60,61] In cases of closed injury, midaxial incisions can be used to secure the tendon graft to the bone, avoiding the need for a volar approach and circumferential dissection. Although this technique avoids the theoretical risks associated with looped reconstructions (bony necrosis along the undersurface of the loop and extensor mechanism hindrance), it may cause foreign body reactions to the anchor[62] and is weaker than a double loop reconstruction in cadaveric study.[61]

POSTOPERATIVE CARE AND REHABILITATION

The postoperative care and rehabilitation after flexor pulley reconstruction is not well-defined

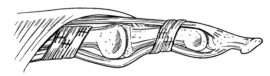

Fig. 4. Completed looped reconstruction of flexor pulley. Copyright Aaron Daluiski, MD; with permission.

and mainly relies on the individual preferences of the surgeon. Okutsu and coworkers[35] recommend a ring-type splint over the proximal phalanx for 14 days following triple-loop reconstruction, whereas Taras and Kaufmann[37] recommend using a ring splint for 6 weeks. Clark and coworkers[8] recommended an intrinsic-plus dorsal blocking splint. Gabl and coworkers[53] and Arora and colleagues[23] place patients in a splint from the proximal palmar crease to the DIP joint, immobilizing the MCP and PIP joints in full extension for 4 weeks.

Both Arora and Gabl initiate finger motion therapy at 4 weeks after nonencircling reconstruction.[23,53] Arora recommends full activities after 3 months[23] and Gabl recommends heavy supportive taping for up to 6 months.[53] Okutsu recommends initiation of active flexion and extension exercises on postoperative day 2 after triple-loop reconstruction.[35] Clark and colleagues has provided the most detailed postoperative protocol.[8] Following a triple-loop reconstruction, passive range of motion and place-and-hold exercises are taught to the patient with a dorsal block splint with supportive pulley strap within the first few days after surgery. In patients with an intact underlying flexor tendon, gentle active motion is started and place-and-hold exercises are continued, using another finger to provide palmar support over the reconstructed pulley. The patient is transitioned to a thermoplastic ring support (see **Fig. 2**) at 3 weeks, which replaces the formal splint by 6 weeks and is worn until 12 weeks. Heavier activities are allowed at 12 weeks.

COMPLICATIONS

Reported complications after flexor pulley reconstruction are relatively rare. The surgeon must ensure proper gliding of the tendon within the tendon sheath to minimize the risk of stiffness and poor functional outcomes. The integrity of the pulley system is predictive of good functional results after 2-stage flexor tendon reconstructions,[63] and the importance of establishing appropriate pulley tension cannot be overemphasized. Careful tenolysis at the beginning of the procedure, taking particular care to remove scar tissue between the tendon and bone, is critical.[8] In addition, overtightening of the pulley inhibits finger motion and may promote the development of synovitis[36] and the formation of flexion contractures.[8]

Failure at the interface between graft and remnant pulley rim has been noted in biomechanical investigations of the Weilby reconstruction.[54] Adverse effects on the volar plate and articular cartilage have been reported after the Karev "belt-loop" reconstruction.[57] Hindrance of the

extensor and flexor mechanisms may occur with looped reconstructions. Furthermore, bone resorption and fracture underneath the graft loop has been reported.[59]

CLINICAL OUTCOMES

Though flexor pulley reconstruction is not that rare, there are only 4 series, all retrospective single-center case series, published in English. Moutet and colleagues reported 12 patients (all rock climbers) who underwent a nonencircling reconstruction using extensor retinaculum graft sutured directly into the remnant pulley rims.[24] All patients returned to rock climbing, with only one failing to return to his or her perceived baseline level of ability. In a series of 6 patients at a mean follow-up of 19.5 months, Gabl and colleagues reported improved flexion and pinch strength after a nonencircling graft of extensor retinaculum with periosteum ("periosteal ligamentous ring graft").[53] There was no comparison to the opposite hand. Postoperative magnetic resonance imaging or ultrasound showed an absence of bowstringing in 5 of 6 patients and reduction in bowstringing in the remaining patient. Arora reported the results of 23 patients undergoing either a Gabl-type or Weilby-type of nonencircling reconstruction.[23] At a mean follow-up of 48 months, the 13 patients who underwent the periosteal ligamentous ring graft had a 97% recovery of PIP flexion, 96% recovery of power grip strength, and 100% recovery of pinch grip compared with the opposite side. At a mean follow-up of 57 months, the 10 patients who underwent the Weilby reconstruction had 94% recovery of PIP flexion, 98% recovery of power grip strength, and 100% recovery of pinch strength. Arora and colleagues concluded that successful results can be obtained with both types of nonencircling reconstructions, but because of its technical difficulty, the periosteal ligamentous ring graft was reserved for patients with high levels of physical activity.[23]

In the only published series of looped pulley reconstructions, Okutsu and colleagues reported a 30° improvement in total active motion of the MCP, PIP, and DIP joints and a 10-mm improvement in tip-to-palm distance in 6 patients who underwent a triple-loop reconstruction.[35] The average follow-up period was 21 months. Because of its rarity, flexor pulley reconstruction is challenging to study with ideal clinical research methods. Hand surgeons must rely on their own experience and judgment to place the findings of biomechanical studies, small case series, and expert clinical opinion within the context of their own practices.

SUMMARY

Flexor pulley reconstruction is a challenging surgery. Regardless of the reconstructive technique used, the surgeon should strive to emulate the length, tension, and glide of the native pulley. Although looped reconstructions have been shown to be stronger in biomechanical studies, nonencircling reconstructions can be successful if the native tissue is amenable to graft healing. The clinical literature, although limited, has shown that return to activity and satisfactory results can be obtained after both nonencircling and looped flexor pulley reconstructions.

ACKNOWLEDGMENTS

The authors would like to acknowledge Mike de la Flor, CMI for his illustrations of the surgical techniques.

REFERENCES

1. Cleveland M. Restoration of the digital portion of a flexor tendon and sheath of the thumb. J Bone Joint Surg Am 1933;15:762–5.
2. Doyle JR, Blythe W. The flexor tendon sheath and pulleys: anatomy and reconstruction. In: Hunter JW, Schneider LH, editors. AAOS Symposium on tendon surgery in the hand. St Louis (MO): The CV Mosby Co; 1975. p. 81–7.
3. Hunter JM, Cook JF, Ochiai N, et al. The pulley system. Orthop Trans 1980;4:4.
4. Manske PR, Lesker PA. Palmar aponeurosis pulley. J Hand Surg Am 1983;8:259–63.
5. Doyle JR. Anatomy of the finger flexor tendon sheath and pulley system. J Hand Surg Am 1988; 13:473–84.
6. Lin GT, Amadio PC, An KN, et al. Biomechanical analysis of finger flexor pulley reconstruction. J Hand Surg Br 1989;14:278–82.
7. Seiler JG. Flexor tendon injury – acute injuries. In: Wolfe SW, Hotchkiss RN, Pederson WC, et al, editors. Green's operative hand surgery. 6th edition. Philadelphia: Elsevier: Churchill Livingston; 2011. p. 159.
8. Clark TA, Skeete K, Amadio PC. Flexor tendon pulley reconstruction. J Hand Surg Am 2010;35: 1685–9.
9. Peterson WW, Manske PR, Bollinger BA, et al. Effect of pulley excision on flexor tendon biomechanics. J Orthop Res 1986;4:96–101.
10. Rispler D, Greenwald D, Shumway S, et al. Efficiency of the flexor tendon pulley system in human cadaver hands. J Hand Surg Am 1996;21:444–50.
11. Kwai Ben I, Elliot D. "Venting" or partial lateral release of the A2 and A4 pulleys after repair of zone 2 flexor tendon injuries. J Hand Surg Br 1998;23:649–54.
12. Tang JB. The double sheath system and tendon gliding in zone 2C. J Hand Surg Br 1995;20:281–5.
13. Savage R. The mechanical effect of partial resection of the digital fibrous flexor sheath. J Hand Surg Br 1990;15:435–42.
14. Mitsionis G, Bastidas JA, Grewal R, et al. Feasibility of partial A2 and A4 pulley excision: effect on finger flexor tendon biomechanics. J Hand Surg Am 1999;24:310–4.
15. Tomaino M, Mitsionis G, Basitidas J, et al. The effect of partial excision of the A2 and A4 pulleys on the biomechanics of finger flexion. J Hand Surg Br 1998;23:50–2.
16. Tang JB, Wang YH, Gu YT, et al. Effect of pulley integrity on excursions and work of flexion in healing flexor tendons. J Hand Surg Am 2001;26:347–53.
17. Tang JB, Xie RG, Cao Y, et al. A2 pulley incision or one slip of the superficialis improves flexor tendon repairs. Clin Orthop Relat Res 2007;456:121–7.
18. Franko OI, Lee NM, Finneran JJ, et al. Quantification of partial or complete A4 pulley release with FDP repair in cadaveric tendons. J Hand Surg Am 2011;36:439–45.
19. Bowers WH, Kuzma GR, Bynum DK. Closed traumatic rupture of finger flexor pulleys. J Hand Surg Am 1994;19:782–7.
20. Schoffl VR, Schoffl I. Injuries to the finger flexor pulley system in rock climbers: current concepts. J Hand Surg Am 2006;31:647–54.
21. Tropet Y, Menez D, Balmat P, et al. Closed traumatic rupture of the ring finger flexor tendon pulley. J Hand Surg Am 1990;15:745–7.
22. Lourie GM, Hamby Z, Raasch WG, et al. Annular flexor pulley injuries in professional baseball pitchers: a case series. Am J Sports Med 2011;39:421–4.
23. Arora R, Fritz D, Zimmermann R, et al. Reconstruction of the digital flexor pulley system: a retrospective comparison of two methods of treatment. J Hand Surg Eur 2007;32:60–6.
24. Moutet F, Forli A, Voulliaume D. Pulley rupture and reconstruction in rock climbers. Tech Hand Up Extrem Surg 2004;8:149–55.
25. Kaufmann RA, Pacek CA. Pulley reconstruction using palmaris longus autograft after repeat trigger release. J Hand Surg Br 2006;31:285–7.
26. Martinoli C, Bianchi S, Cotten A. Imaging of rock climbing injuries. Semin Musculoskelet Radiol 2005;9:334–45.
27. Guntern D, Goncalves-Matoso V, Gray A, et al. Finger A2 pulley lesions in rock climbers: detection and characterization with magnetic resonance imaging at 3 tesla–initial results. Invest Radiol 2007; 42:435–41.
28. Parellada JA, Balkissoon AR, Hayes CW, et al. Bowstring injury of the flexor tendon pulley system: MR imaging. AJR Am J Roentgenol 1996; 167:347–9.

29. Klauser A, Frauscher F, Bodner G, et al. Finger pulley injuries in extreme rock climbers: depiction with dynamic US. Radiology 2002;222:755–61.

30. Bollen SR. Injury to the A2 pulley in rock climbers. J Hand Surg Br 1990;15:268–70.

31. Strickland JW. Development of flexor tendon surgery: twenty-five years of progress. J Hand Surg Am 2000;25:214–35.

32. Dona E, Walsh WR. Flexor tendon pulley V-Y plasty: an alternative to pulley venting or resection. J Hand Surg Br 2006;31:133–7.

33. Bunata RE. Primary pulley enlargement in zone 2 by incision and repair with an extensor retinaculum graft. J Hand Surg Am 2010;35:785–90.

34. Messina A, Messina JC. The direct midlateral approach with lateral enlargement of the pulley system for repair of flexor tendons in fingers. J Hand Surg Br 1996;21:463–8.

35. Okutsu I, Ninomiya S, Hiraki S, et al. Three-loop technique for A2 pulley reconstruction. J Hand Surg Am 1987;12(5 Pt 1):790–4.

36. Mehta V, Phillips CS. Flexor tendon pulley reconstruction. Hand Clin 2005;21:245–51.

37. Taras JS, Kaufmann RA. Flexor tendon injury - flexor tendon reconstruction. In: Wolfe SW, Hotchkiss RN, Pederson WC, et al, editors. Green's operative hand surgery. 6th edition. Philadelphia: Elsevier: Churchill Livingston; 2011. p. 159.

38. Lister GD. Reconstruction of pulleys employing extensor retinaculum. J Hand Surg Am 1979;4:461–4.

39. Tang JB, Zhang QG, Ishii S. Autogenous free sheath grafts in reconstruction of injured digital flexor tendon sheath at the delayed primary stage. J Hand Surg Br 1993;18:31–2.

40. Odobescu A, Radu A, Brutus JP, et al. Modified flexor digitorum superficialis slip technique for A4 pulley reconstruction. J Hand Surg Eur 2010;35:464–8.

41. Nishida J, Amadio PC, Bettinger PC, et al. Flexor tendon-pulley interaction after pulley reconstruction: a biomechanical study in a human model in vitro. J Hand Surg Am 1998;23:665–72.

42. Seiler JG, Uchiyama S, Ellis F, et al. Reconstruction of the flexor pulley. The effect of the tension and source of the graft in an in vitro dog model. J Bone Joint Surg Am 1998;80:699–703.

43. Naidu SH, Rinkus K. Multiple-loop, uniform-tension flexor pulley reconstruction. J Hand Surg Am 2007; 32:265–8.

44. Bader KF, Sethi G, Curtin JW. Silicone pulleys and underlays in tendon surgery. Plast Reconstr Surg 1968;41:157–64.

45. Wray RC Jr, Weeks PM. Reconstruction of digital pulleys. Plast Reconstr Surg 1974;53:534–6.

46. Semer NB, Bartle BK, Telepun GM, et al. Digital pulley reconstruction with expanded polytetrafluoroethylene (PTFE) membrane at the time of tenorrhaphy in an experimental animal model. J Hand Surg Am 1992;17:547–50.

47. Bartle BK, Telepun GM, Goldberg NH. Development of a synthetic replacement for flexor tendon pulleys using expanded polytetrafluoroethylene membrane. Ann Plast Surg 1992;28:266–70.

48. Dunlap J, McCarthy JA, Manske PR. Flexor tendon pulley reconstructions–a histological and ultrastructural study in non-human primates. J Hand Surg Br 1989;14:273–7.

49. Oruc M, Ulusoy MG, Kankaya Y, et al. Pulley reconstruction with different materials: experimental study. Ann Plast Surg 2008;61:215–20.

50. Brand PW, Cranor KC, Ellis JC. Tendon and pulleys at the metacarpophalangeal joint of a finger. J Bone Joint Surg Am 1975;57:779–84.

51. Lalonde DH. Wide-awake flexor tendon repair. Plast Reconstr Surg 2009;123:623–5.

52. Klinert HE, Bennett JB. Digital pulley reconstruction employing the always present rim of the previous pulley. J Hand Surg Am 1978;3:297–8.

53. Gabl M, Reinhart C, Lutz M, et al. The use of a graft from the second extensor compartment to reconstruct the A2 flexor pulley in the long finger. J Hand Surg Br 2000;25:98–101.

54. Widstrom CJ, Doyle JR, Johnson G, et al. A mechanical study of six digital pulley reconstruction techniques: part II. Strength of individual reconstructions. J Hand Surg Am 1989;14:826–9.

55. Karev A, Stahl S, Taran A. The mechanical efficiency of the pulley system in normal digits compared with a reconstructed system using the "belt loop" technique. J Hand Surg Am 1987;12:596–601.

56. Karev A. In reply. J Hand Surg Am 1993;18:171–2.

57. Eaton CJ. Possible complication of belt loop pulley reconstruction. J Hand Surg Am 1993;18:169–70.

58. Boyes JH. Bunnell's surgery of the hand. 5th edition. Philadelphia: J B Lippincott Co; 1970.

59. Lin GT. Bone resorption of the proximal phalanx after tendon pulley reconstruction. J Hand Surg Am 1999;24:1323–6.

60. Slesarenko Y. Minimally invasive technique for finger flexor pulley reconstruction. Hand Surg 2006;11:153–7.

61. Mallo GC, Sless Y, Hurst LC, et al. Minimally invasive A2 flexor tendon pulley and biomechanical comparison with two accepted techniques. Tech Hand Up Extrem Surg 2008;12:170–3.

62. Schrumpf MA, Lee AT, Weiland AJ. Foreign-body reaction and osteolysis induced by an intraosseous poly-L-lactic acid suture anchor in the wrist: case report. J Hand Surg Am 2011;36:1769–73.

63. Wehbe MA, Mawr B, Hunter JM, et al. Two-stage flexor-tendon reconstruction. Ten-year experience. J Bone Joint Surg Am 1986;68:752–63.

Tendon Reconstruction with Adjacent Finger Hand Tendon

Laura-Carmen Sita-Alb, MD[a], Sébastien Durand, MD, PhD[b],*

KEYWORDS

- Tendon reconstruction • Hemi tendon transfer • Delayed treatment
- Zone 1 and 2 tendon reconstruction

KEY POINTS

- Delayed presentation of flexor digitorum profundus (FDP) tendon injury is difficult to repair or reconstruct. An ideal treatment is still to be found.
- We propose 2 new techniques for FDP reconstruction that allow immediate postoperative mobilization and can restore function of digital flexion.
- Both hemi-FDP and hemi-flexor digitorum superficialis (FDS) tendon transfers, are the closest match in terms of muscle agonism and excursion, and do not result in an imbalance of forces across the donor joint with the potential complications that this may create.

INTRODUCTION

The delayed presentation or diagnosis of flexor tendon injury usually lead to worse outcomes. Ideal options for these cases remain to be found. For early repair, the primary direct suture, when possible, is the first choice of treatment. Secondary tendon reconstruction is even more difficult and results are generally worse than primary repair. The most difficult areas that have constantly captured the surgeon's attention are the "no man's land" and zone 1.

The delay in flexor tendon treatment is either due to a complex trauma, where primary repair is not possible, or a delayed diagnosis. A simple test can easily make the diagnosis (inability to actively flex the distal interphalangeal [DIP] joint while the proximal interphalangeal [PIP] joint is held in hyperextension gives the diagnosis of the flexor digitorum profundus tendon rupture). In some cases, however, especially for closed avulsion injuries, the diagnosis can be missed.

DELAYED FLEXOR DIGITORUM PROFUNDUS REPAIR OPTIONS

Many techniques have been used to reconstruct the flexor digitorum profundus tendon (FDP); each technique has its applicability. Many factors influence the decision of treatment and also prognosis of these injuries. Some of these factors are

- The time of delay between the accident and the moment of treatment (probably the most important)
- The level of tendon retraction
- The blood supply of the tendon and soft tissue conditions
- The presence or absence of flexor digitorum superficialis (FDS) injury

Management of old injuries left untreated or misdiagnosed is difficult, often resulting in poor outcome.

Quite a few techniques are currently available for treatment. Usually the treatment involves

[a] Plastic Surgery and Reconstructive Microsurgery, Groupe Main Provence, 42 Maréchal de Lattre de Tassigny Street, 13090 Aix-en-Provence, France; [b] Hand Surgery and Peripheral Nerve Surgery, Groupe Main Provence, 42 Maréchal de Lattre de Tassigny Street, 13090 Aix-en-Provence, France
* Corresponding author.
E-mail address: sebastien.durand@utc.fr

Hand Clin 29 (2013) 243–250
http://dx.doi.org/10.1016/j.hcl.2013.02.006
0749-0712/13/$ – see front matter © 2013 Elsevier Inc. All rights reserved.

a long period of time, multiple operations, and long rehabilitation periods. That is why one has to individualize the treatment for each patient according to his or her expectation, special requirements and the necessity of active DIP joint flexion.

The most common options are

1. No treatment
2. Arthrodesis
3. Profundus advancement
4. Tendon grafts—the most widespread method of treatment, with the choice of 1 or 2 stage tendon grafting depending on the conditions of the gliding bed and soft tissue injuries[1]
5. Tendon transfers
6. Other techniques: capsulodesis, tenodesis, etc

The main application for tendon transfer in the upper extremity is peripheral nerve injuries,[2] but there are also other indications. When speaking about tendon injuries, tendon transfers are mostly associated with extensor tendon treatment, but several authors have published their work on flexor tendon reconstruction with the use of a tendon transfer.

PROCEDURE FEASIBILITY
The Hemi FDS Tendon Transfer

The FDS tendon transfer is known mostly for the treatment of spastic paralysis and ischemic contracture, unfortunately with many donor site morbidities.[3] This procedure has been rarely considered except for the reconstruction of flexor pollicis longus.[4]

Schneider and Wehbe[5] proposed FDS transfer for the delayed repair of the FDP in zone 3, with many consecutive tenolyses needed.

Zuber and colleagues, in a cadaver study, observed that all FDS tendons (with the exception of little finger's FDS) can be transferred for the reconstruction of the FDP, and even advanced in the same digit, with a tendon elongation in the forearm, if needed.[6]

The hemi FDS tendon transfer for FDP reconstruction does not sacrifice the whole adjacent finger FDS tendon; the authors use only half of the FDS tendon, leaving the other half in place.

The Hemi FDP Tendon Transfer

Though the FDS tendon transfer has already been a treatment option for the spastic paralysis, flexor pollicis longus reconstruction, and profundus reconstruction, the transfer of a profundus tendon to reconstruct an adjacent injured profundus tendon is a new technique.

The feasibility of FDP repair using only half of the FDP tendon, in cases of late presentation of zone 1 avulsion injuries, has been attested by Elliot and colleagues.[7] In their anatomic and clinical study, they have shown that the hemi FDP has a larger cross-sectional area than the palmaris longus (the FDP has almost 3 times the area of palmaris longus tendon), and they have not experienced any complications or tendon ruptures in their patients (clinical series of 6 cases).

Because no publications could be found in the literature, an anatomic study was undertaken by Durand and colleagues to assess its feasibility.[8]

Anatomic study

In an effort to decrease morbidity and complications and improve outcomes, an anatomic study was done to determine if a neighboring profundus tendon could be used as a donor musculotendinous unit in such late presenting cases.

The findings were that an FDP hemi tendon from a neighbor digit could be used as a FDP transfer to all digits excepting the middle finger (being longer than the rest). The FDP of the middle finger reaches all the digits (**Fig. 1**).

SURGICAL PROCEDURES

As with all tendon transfer procedures, it is a prerequisite that all joints of the digit are supple, and the involved finger has adequate soft tissue coverage. The procedure is performed under wrist block, so that correct tensioning of the transfer can be set during the final stage of the procedure by requesting the patient to flex and extend his or her fingers.

These techniques are done in 1 or 2 stages with 3 months apart, with insertion of a silicone rod at first, and obligatory physiotherapy during this interval.

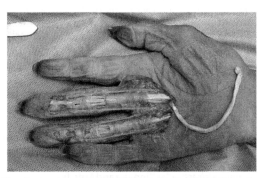

Fig. 1. Anatomic study. FDP tendon isolated from the middle finger can reach any other fingers.

First Stage

Bruner incisions are made to expose the injured tendon sheath. If the soft tissue scaring is minimal, and there are no other associated lesions, a 2-stage procedure is not needed. Unfortunately, however, many times the flexor tendon sheath is damaged and fibrotic, and before the tendon transfer, the flexor tendon sheath must first be recreated.

For the recreation of the flexor tendon sheath, sometimes one needs to enlarge or reconstruct the A2 and A4 pulleys. If one only needs to enlarge the pulleys, a simple plasty might be sufficient. If complete reconstruction is needed, the authors use a free tendon graft; the most used is the palmaris longus tendon graft.

Then a silicone rod is put in place to recreate the tendon sheath, and the authors attach it distally at the distal FDP tendon stump (if it exists).

Second Stage or Continuing First Stage (if Tendon Sheath Permits)

The hemi FDS tendon transfer

The access is via the same technique of Bruner (**Fig. 2**). In the donor digit (the ring finger), after the tendon sheath is exposed, the medial half of the FDS is approached through A3 pulley and sectioned at the level of insertion (**Fig. 3**). The half split is continued as proximally as needed to obtain a sufficient length, this being usually at the level of proximal palmar crease (**Fig. 4**).

In the recipient finger (the little finger), the authors expose the distal stump of the FDP or the distal part of the silicone rod, and then expose the proximal part of the silicone rod in the palm.

The hemi FDS tendon is passed under the neurovascular bundle, and, with the aid of the silicone rod (at which the distal part of the hemi FDS is attached), through the tendon sheath.

Distally, the tendon is secured with a 3–0 nylon through the nail plate using the rope down technique described by Brown.[9]

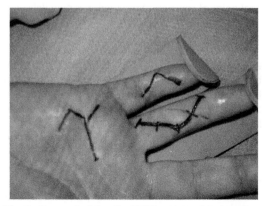

Fig. 2. Bruner incision for FDS hemi tendon transfer.

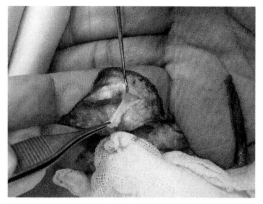

Fig. 3. Sectioning the ulnar half of the FDS of the ring finger at its insertion.

This technique is the authors' favorite, but other techniques for the reinsertion of the FDP are also suitable for insertion of the transferred FDS tendon, such as

- The transosseous suture—the core sutures that reinforce the tendon stump are passed through the distal phalagx, and the ends are tied over a button to the dorsum of the distal phalanx, distal to the lunula to avoid nail deformity[10]; this technique being the most used.
- Profundus pull out through fingertip—in this technique, the core sutures from the tendon are brought out directly to the fingertip, without passing through the bone. This technique is mostly used if a distal stump of the FDP remains.
- The FDP reinsertion using mini-anchors.
- There are also other techniques that combine the previous ones, such as anchor and pull-out through finger tip, or anchor and pull-out to bone technique.

The hemi FDP tendon transfer

The incisions are across the middle and distal phalanges both for the donor and the recipient neighboring digit, with the occasional need of extension up to the distal palmar crease (**Fig. 5**).

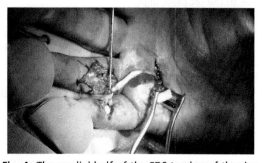

Fig. 4. The medial half of the FDS tendon of the ring finger is ready to be transferred.

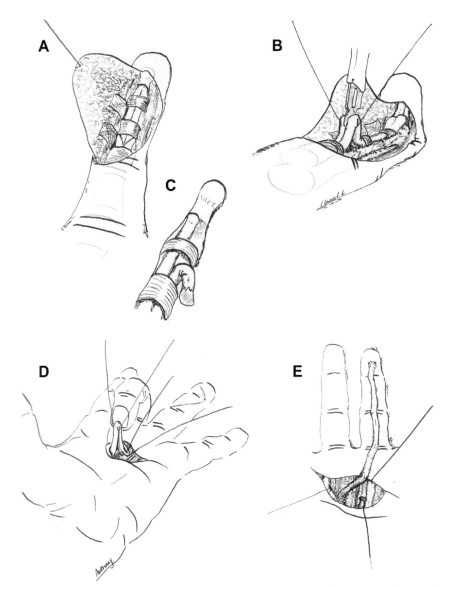

Fig. 5. Technique of hemi-FDP tendon transfer. (*A*) Donor digit incision with opening of C1 and C3 cruciate pulleys. (*B*) Division of FDP into radial and ulnar bundles. (*C*) Disinsertion of hemi tendon. (*D*) The donor FDP is located in the palm (with a sling placed around it), and traction is placed in it in a proximal direction so that the donor digit is placed in maximal flexion. The proximal point of splitting of the tendon is now delivered into the palm, and the whole donor hemi tendon retrieved from the fibroosseous sheath. (*E*) Transfer of the hemi FDP to the recipient digit.

The recipient digit is prepared at first; the authors identify the distal stump of FDP tendon (if present) and the pulley system. The distal stump of the FDP is then excised and a periosteal window created with the cortex of the phalanx being roughened. The palmar incision is then made and the proximal stump of the FDP identified and then divided as proximally as possible under tension.

In the donor digit, the volar groove in the FDP tendon is identified in zone 1 of the flexor sheath,

and the tendon is gently pared into radial and ulnar bundles using a scalpel. Attention is then turned to the insertion of the tendon, and the hemi tendon that borders the recipient digit is divided at its insertion into the terminal phalanx.

The selected hemi tendon is delivered into the palm by traction; then the tendon is further split in proximal, care being taken not to damage the musculotendinous unit in any way.

Then the donor tendon is passed superficially to the lumbrical tendon and deep to the neurovascular bundle, to the A1 pulley of the recipient digit. The hemi tendon is secured to the nail plate with a 3/0 prolene suture after adjustment of tension. Immediate controlled active mobilization of all digits is performed.

Postoperative Care

Postoperatively, a dorsal splint is applied to the hand with the wrist and fingers at 45° of flexion for 3 weeks with immediate controlled active mobilization of the digits.

CLINICAL EXPERIENCE
The Hemi FDS Tendon Transfer

The authors performed the hemi FDS tendon transfer in 2 patients with old FDP tendon ruptures of the little fingers. The authors chose the medial half of the ring finger FDS.

At 3 months, the 2 patients had almost complete flexion and extension in the little fingers, with tip-to-palm distance of 0 mm, and no donor site morbidities (**Fig. 6**A, B).

Even though cadaveric studies indicate the feasibility of FDS tendon transfer for all digits FDP reconstructions (with the exception of little finger FDS) and the advancement of the FDS tendon in the same digit for FDP reconstruction,[6] no clinical trials support that this procedure is better than existing methods. The authors' experience is limited only to the reconstruction of the little finger. Theoretically, however, it is possible to use the hemi FDS tendons (excepting the little finger FDS tendon) to reconstruct an adjacent FDP.

The authors recommend the hemi FDS tendon transfer for little finger FDP reconstruction, but they feel that further clinical studies are needed to confirm no donor site morbidities.

The Hemi FDP Tendon Transfer

The hemi FDP tendon transfer was performed in 4 patients who had not had any other treatment. The site of injury was zone 1 in 2 cases and zone 2 in the other 2 cases. The transfers were performed at a mean of 5 months (range 3–12 months) from injury.

All patients regained good active movement in the DIP joint. There was donor site morbidity in 1 finger with 50° loss of active flexion in the DIP joint. This complication is related, in the authors' view, to the delay of rehabilitation due to pain mismanagement (**Fig. 7**A, B).

The authors consider that this technique can be an option for the delayed treatment of profundus lesions, when direct suture (without extensive flexion deformity) cannot be performed.

DISCUSSIONS
The Hemi FDS Tendon Transfer

Using only half of the FDS, some might say that it is a too thin graft, but if one compares it with the palmaris longus graft, they have approximately the same size, and the FDP of the little finger is also thinner than the other FDP.

Advantages

The type of tendon graft may affect the outcomes of secondary tendon repair. It was demonstrated that an intrasynovial donor graft gives greater mobility and less adherence formation than an extrasynovial tendon graft.[11] Also the utility of vascularized tendon grafts may be even better for functional recovery.

The authors find that hemi FDS tendon graft has several advantages. The muscle has approximately the similar architectural characteristics,

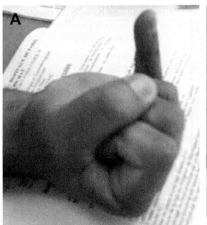 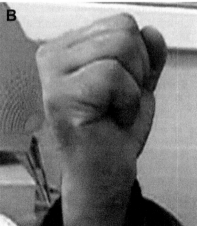

Fig. 6. (*A*) Patient with FDP and FDS traumatic lacerations, before hemi FDS tendon transfer. (*B*) Patient at 4 months after hemi FDS tendon transfer from the ring finger, with complete flexion of the little finger.

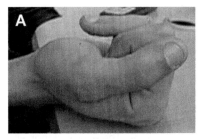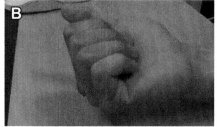

Fig. 7. (*A*) Patient with fourth finger FDP avulsion. (*B*) Patient at 6 months after hemi FDP tendon transfer from the middle finger.

similar force, and similar potential excursion as FDP.[6] Additionally, it is an intrasynovial and a vascularized graft; it has the needed length for reconstructing the little finger's FDP without using a tendon advancement technique.

Complications

When the whole FDS is used for different tendon reconstruction techniques, the donor site complications can become important. Long-term follow-up after superficialis transfer for intrinsic muscle replacement has demonstrated the potential donor site morbidity. Potential complications include swan-neck deformity of the digit, isolated DIP flexion, check-rein deformity, and reduction in the total arc of finger flexion. The incidence of 1 of the mentioned deformities occurring following FDS harvest has been reported as up to 70%.[3]

The authors use only half of the FDS of the ring finger, so the donor site morbidities (if exist), are minor; the scars are only in the palm. In this series of patients, the authors did not find notable morbidities and donor fingers had good function.

The Hemi FDP Tendon Transfer

The hemi FDP tendon have been used in primary FDP tendon repair.[8] FDP lengthening by tenotomy at the musculotendinous junction has been described for contractures that developed after the repair of FDP.[12]

This lengthening was performed in the second stage, when the repair the digit developed a flexion deformity.[12] This technique was originally devised for delayed primary repair of the flexor pollicis longus (FPL) tendon, although the unique anatomic attributes of the FPL musculotendinous unit (the FPL is a separate muscle, while the FDP has a common muscle belly) may make it more suited for this technique.[13] There is little in the literature regarding its application to the lacerated profundus tendon.

Advantages

The authors feel that their method has a few advantages (**Box 1**).

These advantages stem from the anatomic and physiologic properties of the FDP that have been already recognized by others.[7,14–16] The division of the profundus tendon into radial and ulnar bundles is well recognized.[14–16] Beyond the level of the mid-middle phalanx, the bundles are distinct but connected by peritenon,[15] and a previous article by Elliot and colleagues[7] confirms the feasibility of separating them surgically.

The strength of the FDP hemi tendon is enough according to Elliot and colleagues,[7] not only in the results of their clinical series (no complications or tendon ruptures experienced in 6 cases), but also in the anatomic study showing the relative cross-sectional areas of the FDP and palmaris longus tendons. It seems that the hemi FDP is more than adequate in terms of cross-sectional area compared with a standard plamaris longus tendon graft, and it is capable of withstanding the physiologic loads through the graft. Furthermore the authors found no difficulty in immediate mobilization of their repairs.

A further benefit of the utilization of the hemi tendon is, again as reasoned by Elliot,[7] the smaller diameter structure is easier to fit beneath the

---

Box 1
Advantages of hemi FDP tendon transfer

1. Only one suture site in the tendon
2. The same anatomic and physiologic properties
3. The anatomic division of FDP into radial and ulnar bundles
4. The size of hemi FDP is bigger than the palmaris longus tendon
5. Less adhesions formation
6. Early mobilization is possible
7. Vascularized graft
8. Intrasynovial graft
9. No tendon advancement
10. No scars in the forearm

pulleys of the digital sheath. In their experience, they have been obliged to use a silicone rod in only 1 case, where soft tissue damage was extensive enough to have caused widespread scarring of the pulley system. In all other cases, although the pulleys may have shrunk, they all allowed function of the hemi tendon without restriction.

The passage of the tendon through the FDS chiasma posed no difficulty, and postoperative results demonstrated no compromise of function of with preservation of the superficialis. Preservation of the FDS is another positive factor.[17]

The donor unit is not only the best agonist muscle possible but also an exact match in terms of tendon excursion.[15,16,18] This hemi tendon also has nutrition from its proximal part.[19]

Disadvantages

A major limitation is the inability of its application to the middle finger, because the middle finger is too long to be reached by the adjacent tendons. However, the ring and then little fingers most commonly have avulsion injuries of the FDP tendon (the ring finger being involved in up to 75% of cases).[1,7,20]

SUMMARY

Whether it is a primary or a delayed FDP repair, no general consent has been found, and no perfect treatment has been imposed, stimulating surgeons to constantly improve surgical techniques.

The authors utilized 2 new techniques for FDP reconstruction that allow immediate postoperative mobilization and good functional recovery. Harvesting of the donor hemi tendon, both FDP and FDS, is the closest match in terms of muscle agonism and excursion, and does not result in an imbalance of forces across the donor joint with potential complications.

Even though the hemi FDP tendon transfer can be used only in the index, ring, and little fingers, and the hemi FDS only in the little finger (other studies suggest that it can be used in all digits, but the authors have no experience in this area), the authors believe that these techniques will serve as useful additions to the armamentarium of hand surgeons.

REFERENCES

1. Tuttle H, Olvey S, Stern P. Tendon avulsion injuries of the distal phalynx. Clin Orthop Relat Res 2006;445: 157–68.
2. Gutowski KA. Hand II: Periferal nerves and tendon transfers. Selected Readings in Plastic Surgery 2003;9(33):1–55.
3. Brandsma J, Jonge MO. Flexor digitorum superficialis tendon transfer for intrinsic replacement. J Hand Surg Br 1992;17:625–8.
4. Posner MA. Flexor superficialis tendon transfers to the thumb—an alternative to the free tendon graft for treatment of chronic injuries within the digital sheath. J Hand Surg Am 1983;8:876–81.
5. Schneider L, Wehbe M. Delayed repair of flexor profundus tendon in the palm (zone 3) with superficialis transfer. J Hand Surg Am 1988;13:227–30.
6. Zuber C, Della Santa DR, Gajisin S. Replacement of flexor digitorum profundus tendons by transfer of flexor superficialis tendons. An anatomical study. Ann Chir Main Memb Super 1997;16: 235–44.
7. Elliot D, Khandwala A, Ragoowansi R. The flexor digitorum profundus "demi-tendon"—a new technique for the passage of the flexor profundus tendon through the A4 pulley. J Hand Surg Br 2001;26: 422–6.
8. Durand S, Oberlin C, Macquillan A. FDP to FDP hemi-tendon transfer—a new technique for delayed repair of the flexor digitorum profundus in zones I and II of the finger. J Hand Surg Eur 2010;35: 677–8.
9. Marin Braun F, Foucher G, Buchjaeger N, et al. Repair of the flexor digitorum profundus and the flexor pollicis longus by the "rope down" technique. Results in a series of 77 cases. Ann Chir Main Memb Super 1991;10:13–21.
10. Strickland JW. Flexor tendons: acute injuries. In: Green DP, Hotchkiss RN, Pederson WC, editors. Green's operative hand surgery. 4th edition. New York: Churchill Livingstone; 1999. p. 1851–97.
11. Leversedge FJ, Seiler JG 3rd. Flexor digitorum profundus tendon grafting (intrasynovial donor tendons). Oper Tech Orthop 1998;8:106–15.
12. LeViet D. Flexor tendon lengthening by tenotomy at the musculotendinous junction. Ann Plast Surg 1986;17:239–46.
13. Rouhier G. Restoration of the long flexor of the thumb without sacrificing the primary tendon. J Chir (Paris) 1950;66:537–42.
14. Martin B. The tendons of flexor digitorum profundus. J Anat 1958;92:602–8.
15. Goodman H, Choueka J. Biomechanics of flexor tendons. Hand Clin 2005;21:129–49.
16. Grewal R, Sotereanos D, Rao U, et al. Bundle pattern of the flexor digitorum profundus tendon in zone II of the hand: a quantitative assessment of the size of a laceration. J Hand Surg Am 1996;21: 978–83.
17. Strickland J. Delayed treatment of flexor tendon injuries including grafting. Hand Clin 2005;21: 219–43.
18. Brunelli F, De Bellis U, Papalia I, et al. An anatomical study of the relationship between excursion of the

flexor tendons and digital mobility: proposition of an intraoperative test for flexor tendon tenolysis. Surg Radiol Anat 2001;23:243–8.

19. Kessler F. Use of a pedicled tendon transfer with a silicone rod in complicated secondary flexor tendon repairs. Plast Reconstr Surg 1972;49: 439–43.

20. Leddy J, Packer J. Avulsion of the profundus tendon insertion in athletes. J Hand Surg Am 1977;2:66–9.

Outcomes and Evaluation of Flexor Tendon Repair

Jin Bo Tang, MD

KEYWORDS

- Flexor tendon • Primary repair • Secondary repair • Outcomes • Assessment criteria
- Level of expertise of the surgeons

KEY POINTS

- Most reports document a good or excellent recovery of the function of the repaired digits of more than about 80% from fine hand units over recent years, but outcomes in general hospital settings can be more disappointing.
- Over recent years, although rupture of the primarily repaired flexor tendons is still seen in the reports, a few have reported not having ruptures after strong surgical repair, judicious venting of the pulley, and early active postoperative tendon motion.
- The Strickland criteria remain the most commonly used to record the outcomes.
- The author proposes modifying the assessment criteria by setting more stringent "excellent" results as recovery to or greater than 90% of the normal finger motion range and by adding "failure" to designate those digits of recovery of active range of motion less than 30%.
- The outcomes should be provided by subzones of the tendon injuries, and the level of expertise of the surgeons is reported to allow comparisons of the results.

Outcomes of flexor tendon repair are associated with (1) total range of active motion of joints, (2) rate of repair ruptures, and (3) severity of flexion or extension deficits. Outcomes of primary flexor tendon repair have improved over the past 30 years.[1–5] However, reports of series of cases of primary digital flexor tendon repair without ruptures of the repair have emerged only very recently, indicating a leap forward toward the goal of no rupture in primary repairs. In recent years, few original reports can be found regarding outcomes of secondary reconstruction, and the outcomes have not greatly changed in several decades.

OUTCOMES DOCUMENTED OVER THE PAST 10 YEARS

The outcomes of primary flexor tendon repair between 1989 and 2004 were reviewed in an article in *Hand Clinics* in 2005.[5] In this article, the information on outcomes with reports from recent years is supplemented. Most recent reports of primary repair in the digital area are regarding 4-strand or 6-strand tendon repairs, made with newer repair techniques.[6–12]

Outcome Reports from Individual Units

In 2008, *The Journal of Hand Surgery (European Volume)* published a series of reports on flexor tendon repairs using 4-strand or 6-strand core tendon sutures combined with early active flexion exercise (**Table 1**).[6–8] These reports indicate lower rupture rates among tendons with strong core tendon repairs, but it has not always been possible to avoid repair ruptures. Caulfield and colleagues[6] reported 416 tendons repaired with a 4-strand Strickland core suture in zones 1 to 4 in 272 patients and obtained 74% good or excellent grades by the Strickland criteria, with only 2% repair ruptures. Hoffmann and colleagues[7] reported 51 fingers of 46 patients with zone 2 flexor

---

Department of Hand Surgery, The Hand Surgery Research Center, Affiliated Hospital of Nantong University, 20 West Temple Road, Nantong 226001, Jiangsu, China
E-mail address: jinbotang@yahoo.com

hand.theclinics.com

Table 1
Large case series of flexor tendon repair and controlled early active motion in the last 8 years

Authors, Year	Number of Digits	Zones	Core Suture Methods	Results[a]	Rupture Rate
Caulfield et al,[6] 2008	416	1–4	4-strand Strickland	74%	2%
Hoffmann et al,[7] 2008	51	2	6-strand Lim/Tsai	78%	2%
	26	2	2-strand Kessler	43%	11%
Navali & Rouhani,[8] 2008	16 (children)	2	6-strand Strickland	94%	0%
	16 (children)	2	2-strand Kessler	88%	6%
Giesen et al,[14] 2009	50	1, 2	6-strand Tang	78% (White) 82% (Buck-Gramcko)	0%
Moehrlen et al,[10] 2009	40	1–3	2-strand M Kessler	92.5%	0%
Trumble et al, 2009	119	2	4-strand Strickland	—	3%
Sandow & McMahon,[12] 2011	73	1, 2	4-strand cruciate	71%	4.6%

[a] Good and excellent rate by Strickland criteria except those given in parentheses.

tendon repair using the 6-strand Lim/Tsai method. Postoperatively, the fingers were moved with a combined Kleinert and Duran early motion regime and place-and-hold exercises. They had 1 (2%) tendon rupture of 51 flexor digitorum profundus (FDP) tendons. Two (4%) fingers required tenolysis. In contrast, in the cases they treated with the 2-strand modified Kessler method, they had repair ruptures in 3 fingers (11%) and tendon adhesions, or dehiscence, in 3 fingers (11%), which required secondary surgery. The good or excellent outcome rate was 78% with the Lim/Tsai method and 43% with the 2-strand Kessler method. Navali and Rouhani[8] reported 32 flexor tendon repairs in zone 2 of 29 children using either the 2-strand modified Kessler method (16 tendons) or the 4-strand Strickland method (16 tendons). They had one rupture and one fair outcome among the tendons with the 2-strand repair, and one fair outcome after the 4-strand repair. Good or excellent outcomes were achieved in other fingers.

In children, repairs of flexor tendons have generally good or excellent results. Early motion exercise is not essential for a tendon to regain a good range of active motion. These observations were further validated in reports by Elhassan and colleagues[9] in 2006 and by Navali and Rouhani[8] in 2008. More recently, in 2009, Moehrlen and colleagues[10] reported results of 49 flexor tendon repair in 39 children using a 2-strand modified Kessler technique. Children underwent an age-adapted early active tendon mobilization. No ruptures of the repair were found. Among 40 fingers assessed according to the Strickland criteria, 29 (72.5%) were excellent, 8 (20%) were good, 3 (7.5%) were fair, and none were poor. All 7 thumbs had excellent results. Moehrlen and

colleagues[10] concluded that good results and very low complication rates can be expected in children, provided extra care is taken in the early tendon mobilization.

In 2009, Trumble and colleagues[11] reported a multicenter prospective randomized trial of zone 2 flexor tendon injuries in 119 digits of 103 patients conducted between 1996 and 2002 to examine the effect of early active motion and passive motion. The tendons were repaired using a 4-strand Strickland suture and a running epitendinous suture. They found significantly greater range of digital motion, smaller digital flexion contractures, and greater patient satisfaction in the active motion group than in the passive motion group. Factors leading to poor results included associated nerve injury, multiple digit injuries, and smoking. Patients treated by a certified hand therapist had better motion and less contracture. Repaired tendons in 2 digits in each group ruptured. This prospective study supports the combination of multistrand tendon repair and early active motion in zone 2 flexor tendon repairs.

In 2011, Sandow and McMahon[12] reported 73 zone 1 and 2 FDP lacerations in 53 patients repaired with a 4-strand single cross-grasp repair technique made with 3-0 braided polyester suture. After active tendon motion exercise, 71% of fingers achieved a good or excellent outcome, with 3 (4.6%) tendon ruptures.

In 2012, Starnes and colleagues[13] analyzed results of zone 2 flexor tendon repairs in 2 groups: sharp injury group (24 fingers in 21 patients) and saw injury group (17 fingers in 13 patients), performed between 2001 and 2010. The cases with digital fractures were not included. The FDP tendons were repaired with a minimum of a 4-strand core suture technique except that one patient in the saw group had incomplete information. In the saw injury group, 9 of 14 fingers with a 50% or greater laceration of FDS tendon were repaired; in the sharp laceration group, 15 of 18 such FDS injuries were repaired. The saw group had significantly less total range of active and passive motion of the fingers compared with the sharp group. There was no significant difference in grip strength of the hand. Tendons in one finger ruptured in the saw group; none ruptured in the sharp group. Tenolysis was required in 4 of 17 fingers in the saw group and 3 of 24 fingers in the sharp group.

Two recent reports documented no repair rupture using strong tendon repairs, pulley-venting, and early active tendon motion. In 2009 Giesen and colleagues[14] reported outcomes of repair of 50 flexor pollicis longus tendons with Tang's triple Tsuge repair between 2004 and 2008. No peripheral stitches were added after core suture. They reported excellent or good results in 78% of the cases using White criteria or 82% of the cases using Buck-Gramcko criteria. No repair rupture was found in this series. In 2011, Al-Qattan[15] reported repair of zone 2A and 2B FDP tendons with the "figure of eight" 6-strand suture technique in a series of 36 patients (36 fingers) with clean-cut isolated FDP tendon injuries. The pulleys proximal to the tendon laceration level were vented. Postoperatively, early active exercises were performed. There were no ruptures and a good recovery of range of finger motion.

Venting the narrow part of a major pulley is usually achieved through direct incision of a part of the pulley. Other methods besides direct incision have been used. In 2005 Bakhach and colleagues[16] reported expanding the volume of the A2 or A4 pulleys (ie, omega pulley plasty) in 12 patients to allow freer tendon gliding. Through a lateral incision on the junction site of the sheath and periosteum, they released lateral attachment of the pulley and underneath the periosteum over the phalanx, but did not reach inside the sheath. Although most of the patients had good recovery of active digital flexion, 7 fingers required tenolysis. In 2010, Bunata[17] presented results of zone 1 and 2 tendon repair in 9 fingers (7 patients) with a 2-strand modified Kessler and a running circumferential suture. The entire A2 or A4 pulleys were enlarged by incision and repaired with an interposed extensor retinaculum graft, because tendon repair in these cases failed to glide smoothly and without snagging through the tight-fitting pulleys. By the Strickland criteria, there were 3 excellent results, 2 good results, 2 fair results, and 2 poor results. There were no tendon ruptures, but 2 fingers required tenolysis and 2 had bowstringing. It is noteworthy that some of

Bakhach's cases needed tenolysis, and 2 among Bunata's cases had bowstringing and one had tenolysis, indicating drawbacks of these plasty procedures. The complex plasty may increase adhesions; the plasty over the entire length of the A2 pulley may cause tendon bowstringing. In our unit, the author does not perform plasty and considers venting by means of a simple incision sufficient; the venting should not involve the entire A2 pulley.

Over the last decade, few reports have been made on the outcomes of secondary repair. It is assumed that the outcomes of secondary tendon graft reconstruction or staged reconstruction have not been changed since reports of several decades ago.

Meta-Analysis of the Outcomes

In 2012, Dy and colleagues[18] presented a meta-analysis of complications associated with flexor tendon repair. After extracting demographics, zone of injury, core suture technique (only modified Kessler or a combination of techniques), use of epitendinous suture, and date of publication (before or after January 1, 2000), unadjusted meta-analysis revealed rates of reoperation of 6%, rupture of 4%, and adhesions of 4%. Meta-regression analysis of 29 studies showed that core suture technique or use of an epitendinous suture does not influence rupture. Although complication rates were generally low, their data suggest no definitive changes in complication rates when repaired before 2000 than after 2000.

The decrease of the rupture rates has been seen to decrease in reports of more recent years, typically after 2005. Division of treatment period into before and after 2000 would not reveal this difference in that study. Only modified Kessler and its combination forms were included, which excluded comparison of the low-profile repair methods with the high-profile methods. In the report of Dy and colleagues,[18] 4% of the tendons developed adhesions that necessitated tenolysis. The rate of formation of adhesions around the repaired tendon should be higher than 4%. Adhesions usually occur in most repaired tendons, varying in their severity and some not hampering tendon motion.

DISCREPANCIES BETWEEN REPORTED OUTCOMES AND THOSE FROM MORE GENERAL SETTINGS

Reports of primary flexor tendon repair and some secondary reconstruction procedures documented good outcomes, but in a general setting, more disappointing cases are seen than are read about in the literature. No articles have specifically addressed this discrepancy, but the reasons may include the following:

1. The results of primary repair or secondary reconstruction have mostly come from hand centers with experienced or master surgeons on the team.
2. Surgeons tend not to make reports based on case series whereby more disappointing results are seen than other reports.
3. The surgical team and rehabilitation setup are not ideal, and practice guidelines or knowledge may not have been updated. The surgeons are aware that their suboptimal results stem from such conditions and think that making such reports would contribute nothing meaningful to the literature.
4. Current clinical outcome reports are based mainly on simple injuries, chiefly involving the laceration of tendons (and adjacent nerves), but clinically more severe injuries are encountered. Outcomes of tendon repair after complex injuries have rarely been reported.

If a repair is performed by an inexperienced surgeon (including trainees or surgeons who do not often deal with tendon repair), one who does not abide by general guidelines for tendon repair, one who has not kept up-to-date on the key issues of correct surgery, or one who practices in a unit without established postoperative care, there will be a high incidence of poor functional return, disruption of the repair, and severe finger stiffness. It is important to update surgery and postoperative care to optimize the outcomes of tendon repair. Frequently, even if the surgeons and therapists keep their knowledge up-to-date, there may be a discrepancy between what they read and how they can apply that knowledge.

The problems that should be dealt with properly with during surgery and in the early and late periods after surgery are summarized in **Fig. 1**.

Nowadays, fewer cases require secondary reconstruction than primary repair. If secondary tendon reconstruction is required for a patient, trauma to the hand of the patient is usually more severe, because (1) the tendon defect may be associated with severe hand trauma, which leads to more complex injuries involving multiple tissues; or (2) secondary repair is indicated for cases unsuitable for primary repair, including tendon bed scar and destruction of the pulley system.

KEYS FOR SUCCESSFUL REPAIRS: PRIMARY AND SECONDARY
Attention to the Details of Techniques: Quality of Surgery, Tension, and Others

Attention to the technical details of surgery is the most important consideration for tendon surgery in the hand. Atraumatic handling is an essential approach to the tendon. Understanding the biomechanics of the tendon and surgical repair is essential to successful surgery and rehabilitation.[19] Many decisions are made based on a deep understanding of tendon mechanics and according to actual situations seen on the operating table. Tension should always been a concern whenever a surgeon performs a direct repair or grafting.[20] In primary repair, tension over the entire tendon should be as low as possible, but tension across the repair sites (in the segment encompassed by the core sutures) should be higher to resist gapping. In tendon grafting, tension should be maintained across the grafted tendon during surgery, because some elasticity of the muscle belly will return postoperatively, decreasing the tension originally set through the graft.

Strong Tendon-bone Attachment, End-to-end Repair, and Proximal Junction

"Strong" repairs are a requirement for all tendon procedures. The method of rebuilding the tendon-bone junction is now undergoing a transition from

Clinical Problems in Primary Flexor Tendon Repairs

During Surgery	Early After Surgery	Late After Surgery
• Handling of tendon • Surgical quality • Treatment judgment	• Repair gapping during motion • Repair caught in pulley rims • Swollen tendon get stuck, unable to glide • Pain and swelling prevent digital motion	• Finger joint stiffness • Adhesion formation • Loss of smooth tendon surface

Fig. 1. The problems that surgeons have to deal with during surgery of primary repair, and in the early and late postoperative periods. The tendon injuries in the little fingers are sometimes particularly difficult to treat.

the pull-out suture to the newer no-button methods. Adequate mechanical strength is required for the newer methods for the tendon-bone attachment. The interweaving suture technique has been a standard and reliable way to complete a proximal junction of tendon grafting. All end-to-end tendon repairs should be mechanically sound. The driving force behind the increasing popularity of strong surgical repair is to avoid rupture of the repair in the first few weeks after surgery—at this time, the biologic tendon healing has not yet translated to a gain in mechanical strength of the tendon, so the surgical repair strength acts primarily to resist gapping or rupture of the repair. Recent development allows use of stronger sutures, such as Fiberwire (Arthrex, North Naples, FL),[21] and of stronger repair methods, with greater care for surgical details, which act in concert to ensure a mechanically sound surgical repair.[19,22]

Attention to the Diameter of the Pulleys and How the Tendon Fits into the Pulleys

Treatment of pulleys has been a major focus of discussion in primary repair. Partial venting of the A2 pulley is effective in allowing greater degrees of tendon motion and will not lead to bowstringing if the other annular pulleys are intact and total release of the sheath-pulley is less than 2 cm.

During secondary surgery, dealing with pulleys properly is equally important. If multiple annular pulleys are damaged, reconstructed pulleys should be strong and properly located at the A2 and A4 sites. The A2 pulley can be vented partly to allow tendon motion during tenolysis, provided most of the sheath is intact. In all tendon surgery, surgeons should consider the diameters of the pulleys and how the tendon fits inside them. It is crucial to always leave room to accommodate edema and swelling of tendons that have been operated on.

Use the Extension-flexion Test to Assure That a Repair is Appropriate for Early Active Motion

The author recommends that the surgeon always perform a simple but important test, what the author calls the "extension-flexion test", to verify tension across the repair site and strength of the repair. This simple test should be performed immediately after surgical tendon repair and sheath-pulley venting are completed. The test consists of 3 parts (**Fig 2**). Step 1: full extension of the repaired digit to observe whether gapping occurs at the repair site. Step 2: mild to moderate flexion of the digit to observe whether the tendon can passively glide. And Step 3: marked or full flexion of the digit to observe whether the repair site of the tendon (or core suture knots, peripheral sutures) impinge

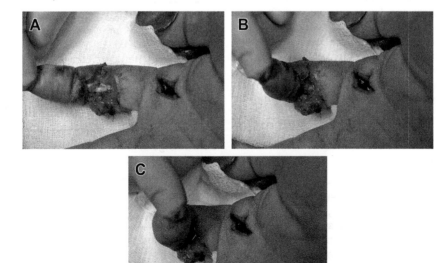

Fig. 2. The digital "extension-flexion test" consists of three parts. (*A*) Step 1: to make sure gapping does not occur at the repair site at full extension of the repaired digit. (*B*) Step 2: make sure that the tendon glides in the range of mild to moderate flexion of the digit. (*C*) Step 3: make sure the repair site and suture knots do not impinge upon the rim of the proximal sheath-pulley when the digit is moved to marked (or full) digital flexion. The repair should pass each of these steps before surgeon proceeds to closure of surgical incision. The surgeon should redo the repair if failed to pass the test.

upon the rim of the proximal sheath-pulley. The repair should "pass" each of these steps before surgeon proceeds to closure of skin incision. If the repair fails the test, the surgeon should either redo the repair to eliminate gapping at the repair site or ensure that the proximal sheath-pulley no longer catches the repair site. Actively extending and flexing the repaired fingers to check each above step during wide-awake surgery would provide even clearer assessment of the repair. The surgeon should clearly document the findings during the test—pass, failed, or gapping, catching—into the surgical chart, and properly inform the therapists with results of this intra-operative test. It appears that this method has been used by at least a few of the leading surgeons in this field. However, now it is time to standardize this test and to make it a necessary part of the surgery and documentation. It is hard to imagine that a repair that cannot tolerate the intra-operative extension-flexion test could tolerate early active tendon motion when the surgical incision is closed and edema develops after surgery.

Incorporation of Early Active Motion into Exercise Regime

Early tendon mobilization has been gradually extended into motion regimes after secondary repair. However, most of these regimes are not as aggressive as those after primary repair. It is reasonable to incorporate into the regimes: (1) synergistic wrist and finger motion; and (2) mid-range-only active motion. Both concepts of rehabilitation used after primary repair should be similarly applicable to secondary repair. The lack of strength of reconstructed pulleys, the lengthy skin incisions, and the greater degrees of edema in tendons and other soft tissues prevent very aggressive active tendon motion.

CRITERIA AND DOCUMENTATION OF OUTCOMES
Commonly Used Criteria

The criteria commonly used to evaluate functional recovery, whether after primary repair, delayed primary repair, secondary reconstruction, or tenolysis, is Strickland's original method of 1980 (**Table 2**).[23] Popular use of this method greatly facilitates comparison of outcomes across surgeons, clinics, and geographic areas. The Buck-Gramcko method is probably the second most popular method, used more frequently by German-speaking hand surgeons. The total active range-of-motion method, which includes the motion range of the metacapophaleagel joint,[24] is not popular, and other methods are used only occasionally.

Table 2
Strickland criteria of assessment of functional outcomes of flexor tendon repairs

Function Grade	% Return of Motion[a]
Excellent	85–100 (>150°)
Good	70–84 (125°–149°)
Fair	50–69 (90°–124°)
Poor	0–49 (<90°)

[a] The sum of active ranges of motion of the PIP and DIP joints. % is the comparison to the contralateral side (or 175°). The motion ranges given in parentheses can be used for judgment if the contralateral side is not compared.

Distal Interphalangeal Joint (DIP)-only Criteria for Zone 1 Injury

Moienem and Elliot[25] used a DIP joint-only method to assess the recovery of DIP joint motion after zone 1 tendon repair. This method is in addition to evaluation of either flexor or extensor tendon repair distal to the DIP joint. Use of this method alone would amplify the weight that the DIP joint carries and does not reflect the impact of the tendon injury on the entire digit. Therefore, the criteria are better used in combination with the Strickland criteria, which include both proximal interphalangeal (PIP) and DIP joint active motion.

How to Assess the Range of Finger Motion

In assessing the range of active motion of the fingers, a powerful and persistent grip would produce flexion by as much as 5° to 10° while the range of hand motion is in the process of recovery and some joint stiffness is present. Active flexion range should be measured when the patient comfortably flexes the finger, not after persistent and painful attempts at a greater active range. The measurement is intended to record the active range of motion that is efficient and easy for daily use. The functional evaluation should be finalized after recovery is complete, which may be a year after surgery.

Criteria with More Stringent Scales

Making a more stringent "excellent" category and separately recording the fingers fail to reach 30% return of active range of motion (**Table 3**) are proposed.[26] The method grades the outcomes into excellent, good, fair, poor, and failure categories. These criteria are user-friendly, which can be used to areas other than zone 2. For repairs in zone 2, by this method the overall good to excellent rate is comparable to that in the previous reports using the Strickland criteria.

Table 3
A more stringent criteria of assessment of results of flexor tendon repairs (Tang, 2007)[26]

Function Grade	% Return of Motion[a]
Excellent	90–100
Good	70–89
Fair	50–69
Poor	30–49
Failure	<30

[a] % Total active motion of the contralateral side: for zone 2 injury, only the PIP and DIP joints are included into evaluation. 175° is sum of the motion of the normal PIP and DIP joints.

Data from Tang JB. Indications, methods, postoperative motion and outcome evaluation of primary flexor tendon repairs in zone 2. J Hand Surg Eur 2007;32:118–29.

Strickland used another criteria in 1985,[27] that is considered lenient. The concern about raising the stringency of excellent category has been echoed by other surgeons. Therefore, a more stringent excellent category seems necessary as the results move toward more ideal outcomes.

Inclusion of Report of Level of Expertise

Including a report on the level of expertise of the surgeon is another consideration in reporting outcomes. Results of flexor tendon repairs are expertise-dependent. Unfortunately, the need for reporting expertise is a topic rarely addressed and is not usually included in reports. Flexor tendon repairs are a perfect example of such needs. The need for reporting expertise, however, is not limited to the reports of outcomes of tendon repairs, but extends to many other procedures. Because experience with implemented techniques is not paralleled by job title, simply categorizing surgeons as residents, attending surgeons, or consultants, and so on provides little or no scientific information regarding their expertise in specific techniques. For treatments that rely heavily on proficiency of involved technique, a report of the level of expertise is very beneficial to interpretation of the outcomes. This concept holds particular importance in comparing studies conducted in different institutions or geographic areas.

An example of such criteria is given by which expertise levels of the surgeons who *conduct* the treatment are reported succinctly using a grade, perhaps under "Methods" (**Table 4**).[28] The documented expertise levels are those of the surgeons performing the procedure, rather than the expertise of the senior authors of the report. The expertise levels should also relate to *specific techniques under investigation*, not to the surgeons' overall expertise in practice.

Documentation of Exact Injury Locations

To present clearly to the readers the outcomes of treatment, documenting the sites of tendon injuries

Table 4
Levels of expertise of the surgeons in reporting outcomes of surgical treatment

Levels/Category	Criteria
1. Nonspecialist	A surgeon who is in training or is a general practitioner
2. Specialist—less experienced	A surgeon who has completed training, but who has not yet acquired in-depth knowledge or high-volume experience in the use of the techniques pertinent to the report. Less degree of experience, judged by shorter duration of practice (eg, less than 5 y) as a specialist, or limited exposure to the investigated disorder
3. Specialist—experienced	A surgeon who has obtained sufficient experience in use of the techniques pertinent to the report, practiced as a specialist over a longer period (eg, 5 y or beyond), with reasonably greater exposure to the disorder
4. Specialist—highly experienced	A specialist who possesses in-depth knowledge or treatment experience with use of the relevant techniques This experience is best indicated by having performed, or been involved in, scholastic studies relevant to the disorder or techniques
5. Expert	A highly experienced specialist who has made a recognized contribution to knowledge or treatments related to the disorder being investigated, or who has pioneered the technique in the report

according to refined anatomic nomenclature (eg, subzones of the tendons from the fingertip to the distal palm) is recommended. There are 7 subzones in zones 1 to 2.[25,26] Documentation of injuries and repairs in subzones facilitates interpretation and comparisons of outcomes. Such reports have been seen in recent years.[14,15,29,30]

SUMMARY

Over the past 10 years, surgeons have reported good to excellent results in about 80% or more of the tendons that underwent 4-strand or 6-strand core suture repair, with 2% to 5% repair ruptures. This period saw the first widespread use of multistrand core suture repairs, but in most reports disruption is still seen during early active motion. Reports of no repair rupture in case series have just emerged, suggesting progress toward the goal of primary repair without rupture. The Strickland criteria remain the most common method used to record outcomes. Modifying it by setting a more stringent excellent standard to include only recovery to or greater than 90% of normal finger flexion range and adding a "failure" category to designate cases of functional recovery less than 30% are proposed. Describing the outcomes by subzones of the tendons and reporting the level of expertise of the surgeons offer clear documentation and allow comparisons of the results among different units.

REFERENCES

1. Lister GD, Kleinert HE, Kutz JE, et al. Primary flexor tendon repair followed by immediate controlled mobilization. J Hand Surg Am 1977;2:441–51.
2. Tsuge K, Ikuta Y, Matsuishi Y. Repair of flexor tendons by intratendinous tendon suture. J Hand Surg Am 1977;2:436–40.
3. Small JO, Brennen MD, Colville J. Early active mobilisation following flexor tendon repair in zone 2. J Hand Surg Br 1989;14:383–91.
4. Tang JB, Shi D, Gu YQ, et al. Double and multiple looped suture tendon repair. J Hand Surg Br 1994; 19:699–703.
5. Tang JB. Clinical outcomes associated with flexor tendon repair. Hand Clin 2005;21:199–210.
6. Caulfield RH, Maleki-Tabrizi A, Patel H, et al. Comparison of zones 1 to 4 flexor tendon repairs using absorbable and unabsorbable four-strand core sutures. J Hand Surg Eur 2008;33:412–7.
7. Hoffmann GL, Büchler U, Voeglin E. Clinical results of flexor tendon repair in zone II using a six-strand double-loop technique compared with a two-strand technique. J Hand Surg Eur 2008;33:418–23.
8. Navali AM, Rouhani A. Zone 2 flexor tendon repair in young children: a comparative study of four-strand versus two strand repair. J Hand Surg Eur 2008; 33:424–9.
9. Elhassan B, Moran SL, Bravo C, et al. Factors that influence the outcome of zone I and zone II flexor tendon repairs in children. J Hand Surg Am 2006; 31:1661–6.
10. Moehrlen U, Mazzone L, Bieli C, et al. Early mobilization after flexor tendon repair in children. Eur J Pediatr Surg 2009;19:83–6.
11. Trumble TE, Vedder NB, Seiler JG 3rd, et al. Zone-II flexor tendon repair: a randomized prospective trial of active place-and-hold therapy compared with passive motion therapy. J Bone Joint Surg Am 2010;92:1381–9.
12. Sandow MJ, McMahon M. Active mobilisation following single cross grasp four-strand flexor tenorrhaphy (Adelaide repair). J Hand Surg Eur 2011;36: 467–75.
13. Starnes T, Saunders RJ, Means KR. Clinical outcomes of zone II flexor tendon repair depending on mechanism of injury. J Hand Surg Am 2012;37:2532–40.
14. Giesen T, Sirotakova M, Copsey AJ, et al. Flexor pollicis longus primary repair: further experience with the Tang technique and controlled active mobilization. J Hand Surg Eur Vol 2009;34:758–61.
15. Al-Qattan MM. Isolated flexor digitorum profundus tendon injuries in zones IIA and IIB repaired with figure of eight sutures. J Hand Surg Eur 2011;36: 147–53.
16. Bakhach J, Sentucq-Rigal J, Mouton P, et al. The Omega pulley plasty. A new technique to increase the diameter of the annular flexor digital pulleys. Ann Chir Plast Esthet 2005;50:705–14 [in French].
17. Bunata RE. Primary pulley enlargement in zone 2 by incision and repair with an extensor retinaculum graft. J Hand Surg Am 2010;35:785–90.
18. Dy CJ, Hernandez-Soria A, Ma Y, et al. Complications after flexor tendon repair: a systematic review and meta-analysis. J Hand Surg Am 2012;37:543–51.
19. Tang JB. Flexor tendon repair. In: Neligan P, Chang J, editors. Plastic surgery, Vol. 6. Philadelphia: Elsevier Saunders; 2012. p. 178–205.
20. Wu YF, Tang JB. Effects of tension across the tendon repair site on tendon gap and ultimate strength. J Hand Surg Am 2012;37:906–12.
21. Gan AW, Neo PY, He M, et al. A biomechanical comparison of 3 loop suture materials in a 6-strand flexor tendon repair technique. J Hand Surg Am 2012;37:1830–4.
22. Fufa D, Osei DA, Calfee RP, et al. The effect of core and epitendinous suture modifications on repair of intrasynovial flexor tendons in an in vivo canine model. J Hand Surg Am 2012;37:2526–31.
23. Strickland JW, Glogovac SV. Digital function following flexor tendon repair in zone 2: a comparison of

immobilization and controlled passive motion techniques. J Hand Surg Am 1980;5:537–43.

24. Kleinert HE, Verdan C. Report of the committee on tendon injuries. J Hand Surg Am 1983;8(Suppl): 794–8.

25. Moiemen NS, Elliot D. Primary flexor tendon repair in zone 1. J Hand Surg Br 2000;25:78–84.

26. Tang JB. Indications, methods, postoperative motion and outcome evaluation of primary flexor tendon repairs in Zone 2. J Hand Surg Eur 2007; 32:118–29.

27. Strickland JW. Results of flexor tendon surgery in zone 2. Hand Clin 1985;1:167–79.

28. Tang JB. Re: levels of experience of surgeons in clinical studies. J Hand Surg Eur 2009;34:137–8.

29. Al-Qattan MM. Zone 2 lacerations of both flexor tendons of all fingers in the same patient. J Hand Surg Eur 2011;36:205–9.

30. Dowd MB, Figus A, Harris SB, et al. The results of immediate re-repair of zone 1 and 2 primary flexor tendon repairs which rupture. J Hand Surg Br 2006;31:507–13.

Current Methods and Biomechanics of Extensor Tendon Repairs

Christopher J. Dy, MD, MSPH[a], Lauren Rosenblatt, BS[b],
Steve K. Lee, MD[b],*

KEYWORDS

- Extensor tendon injuries • Extensor tendon repair • Biomechanics
- Running interlocking horizontal mattress

KEY POINTS

- The surgeon should consider the zone of injury when planning suture configuration. The extensor tendons are broad and flat in the distal zones and cannot accommodate core sutures. We prefer the running interlocked horizontal mattress configuration for its technical ease and biomechanical strength.
- It is important for the surgeon to avoid the unintended consequence of joint stiffness, which can occur from prolonged immobilization or inadvertent shortening of the extensor mechanism.
- Although dynamic motion protocols have decreased the frequency of postoperative joint stiffness, the surgeon should carefully balance the risks of joint stiffness and repair rupture during the initial postoperative period.
- Patients should be advised that a slight extensor lag may persist and full finger flexion may not be possible despite seemingly successful treatment, especially in nonacute injuries.

OVERVIEW OF EXTENSOR TENDON INJURIES

Extensor tendon injuries are common, comprising more than one-quarter of orthopedic soft tissue injuries.[1] The combined incidence of extensor tendon disruption and mallet finger injuries is 27.8 cases per 100,000 patients with orthopedic injuries in a well-defined catchment area, ranking ahead of meniscal injuries, Achilles tendon ruptures, and anterior cruciate ligament injuries.[1] The volume of these injuries and their predilection to occur in working-aged patients indicate that extensor tendon injuries contribute greatly to the direct and indirect health care costs to the individual and society.[2,3]

Despite their frequency, extensor tendon injuries do not receive a proportionate amount of attention in the scientific literature. There are noted knowledge gaps and deficiencies in the literature, specifically a paucity of level I evidence to guide the surgical management and postoperative rehabilitation of extensor tendon injuries.[4] There are unique anatomic, biomechanical, and functional considerations that must be kept in mind when treating extensor tendon injuries, making it difficult to adopt principles learned from the extensive study of flexor tendons.

RELEVANT ANATOMY

The hand surgeon must be aware of the numerous variations in the anatomy of the extensor mechanism, such as the extensor carpi radialis intermedius, extensor medii proprius, extensor indices

[a] Department of Orthopaedic Surgery, Hospital for Special Surgery, 535 East 70th Street, New York, NY 10021, USA; [b] Hand and Upper Extremity Service, Department of Orthopaedic Surgery, Hospital for Special Surgery, 535 East 70th Street, New York, NY 10021, USA
* Corresponding author.
E-mail address: leest@hss.edu

Hand Clin 29 (2013) 261–268
http://dx.doi.org/10.1016/j.hcl.2013.02.008

et medii, and extensor digitorum brevis manus.[5] These structures can make the accurate diagnosis of extensor mechanism disorders more challenging, but can also help the hand surgeon as a potential source of tendon grafts.

The extensors reach their musculotendinous junctions 4 cm proximal to the wrist joint, except for the extensor indicis proprius (EIP), whose muscle fibers reach the level of the wrist joint. The extensors are separated into 6 compartments by synovial lined fibro-osseous sheaths as they cross the wrist joint. The extensor retinaculum transversely forms a roof over these compartments and prevents bowstringing of the tendons. In contrast with their round shape within the compartments, the tendons assume a flatter shape as they progress distally into the hand and fingers.

Within the dorsum of the hand, the juncturae tendinae connect the ring extensor digitorum communis (EDC) tendon to the middle and small finger EDC tendons. These stout fibrous bands link the finger extensors together, preventing independent extension of the fingers. The EDC tendons of the index and middle fingers are also connected by a less substantial band. These connections between the finger extensor tendons allow partial maintenance of metacarpophalangeal (MP) joint extension after a laceration of the extensor tendon, provided that the adjacent finger's extensor tendon is still intact and the laceration is proximal to the juncturae tendinae.

As the extensor tendons progress distally to the MP joint, the sagittal bands secure them to the dorsal axial midline. Originating on the volar plate of the MP joint and the intermetacarpal ligaments, these circumferential fibrous thickenings insert along the extensor hood. The sagittal bands allow the extensor tendons to extend the MP joint despite there being no tendinous insertion onto the proximal phalanx. Disruption of the sagittal band, which can occur secondary to open injuries or from chronically acquired laxity, may compromise MP joint extension if the extensor tendons are not maintained in the midline.

Beyond the MP joint, the extensor mechanism becomes more complex. The EDC tendon of each finger trifurcates before reaching the proximal interphalangeal (PIP) joint. The remaining central portion, now referred to as the central slip, crosses the PIP joint and attaches to the middle phalanx. The central slip allows PIP extension. After forming from the intrinsic tendons of the interossei and lumbricals, the lateral bands reach the dorsal portion of the finger at the level of the proximal phalanx. The lateral bands join the remaining radial and ulnar portions from the EDC trifurcation to form the conjoined lateral bands. The conjoined lateral bands proceed distally and cross the distal interphalangeal (DIP) joint before converging to form the terminal tendon, which attaches to the distal phalanx 1.2 mm proximal to the germinal nail matrix.[6]

Balance of the conjoined lateral bands along the dorsal/volar axis of the fingers is essential to maintaining appropriate function of the extensor mechanism at the PIP and DIP joints. The transverse retinacular ligament connects the lateral bands to the volar plate of the PIP joint and prevents them from dorsally subluxating during PIP extension. The triangular ligament connects the conjoined lateral bands over the middle phalanx and prevents them from palmarly subluxating during DIP flexion. Disruption of these stabilizing ligaments can lead to clinically apparent deformities. Boutonnière deformity, with PIP flexion and DIP hyperextension, results from triangular ligament incompetence because the lateral bands migrate volarly. In addition to causing PIP flexion, this increases tension on the conjoined lateral bands and causes DIP hyperextension. Swan neck deformity, with PIP hyperextension and DIP flexion, results from transverse retinacular ligament incompetence. The lateral bands migrate dorsally, resulting in an overpull of extensor force across the PIP joint and a net loss of extension force at the DIP joint.

Zones of Injury

Because the extensor tendons assume a different morphology and level of complexity as they progress from the forearm to the fingers, anatomic classification of these injuries can prove helpful in planning treatment strategies. The anatomic classification most commonly used today was originally described by Kleinert and Verdan,[7] with later modification by Doyle.[8] The zones of injuries progress from zone I at the level of the DIP to zone VII at the wrist joint, with each joint corresponding with an oddly numbered zone. The zones of injury for the thumb are numbered slightly differently because there is only 1 interphalangeal (IP) joint: T1 represents the thumb IP joint and T3 represents the thumb MP joint.

BIOMECHANICAL CONSIDERATIONS

Restoration of appropriate tendon length and excursion is critical in delivering optimal results in the treatment of extensor mechanism injuries. Although the overall tendon excursion of the extensor mechanism is approximately 5 cm, most of this motion occurs proximal to the wrist at the musculotendinous portions. Because only slight excursion occurs in the hand and fingers, even slight changes in tendon length and tension can have undesired effects on finger motion. Over-lengthening of the extensor mechanism, either directly through suboptimal tendon repair tech-nique or indirectly from a fracture, can create an extensor lag. This problem is more pronounced in the fingers because hyperextension of the MP joints can mask an extensor lag in the hand. However, surgeons must be careful not to shorten the extensor tendon, because this can restrict finger flexion. The intricate balance of the extensor mechanism must be maintained to successfully treat these injuries.

Suture Configurations

Although a variety of different suture configura-tions have been described in the treatment of extensor tendon injuries, surgeons should base their treatment on the characteristics of the tendon at the zone of injury. The extensor tendons have a thickness of 1.75 mm along the dorsum of the hand, but narrow to a thickness of 0.65 mm after crossing the MP joint.[8] These broad, flat tendons generally cannot accommodate core sutures, adding to the challenge of providing a repair with appropriate strength and durability. The proximal portions of the extensor tendon are thicker and rounder, allowing them to accommodate core sutures in a manner similar to flexor tendons.

There are few studies on the biomechanics of suture configurations for extensor tendon injuries, particularly compared with flexor tendon injuries. When comparing the biomechanical strength of suture configuration in zones IV and VI, Newport[9] showed the superiority of the Kleinert modification of the Bunnell repair in zone IV and zone VI.[5,9] More recently, Woo and colleagues[10] showed that the modified Becker technique (also referred to as the augmented Becker or Massachusetts General Hospital repair) has greater resistance to gapping, and greater ultimate strength, than a double figure-of-eight, a double modified Kessler, and a 6-strand double loop for zone IV injuries. Howard and colleagues[11] showed the modified Becker technique to be biomechanically superior to a modi-fied Bunnell technique and the Krackow-Thomas technique for zone VI injuries.

In a recent biomechanical study, the senior author compared the modified Bunnell and the modified Becker techniques with a running inter-locked horizontal mattress (R-IHM) suture configu-ration.[12] As its name implies, the R-IHM combines a running suture with an interlocked horizontal mattress suture. The R-IHM was significantly stiffer in ex vivo testing than the modified Bunnell

and modified Becker techniques and also led to less tendon shortening than the other two tech-niques. Furthermore, the R-IHM was significantly quicker to perform than the other two techniques, which specifically addresses a concern raised by Woo and colleagues[10] in their evaluation of the modified Becker/MGH technique. The ultimate strength of the R-IHM suture configuration is 51 N, which permits early motion in situations that demand early mobilization, such as a concom-itant flexor tendon repair.[12] Because of its favor-able biomechanical properties and its technical simplicity for a broad tendon, we think that the R-IHM technique is an ideal suture configuration for extensor tendon repair.

GENERAL TREATMENT CONSIDERATIONS

After being initially evaluated in the emergency department or primary care setting, patients with extensor mechanism injuries should be seen by a surgeon with adequate training in the nonopera-tive and surgical management of these injuries. This assessment ideally occurs within 1 week of the injury. Surgical treatment is generally indicated for patients with greater than 25% laceration of the extensor tendon, those with an inability to extend the finger, those with associated injuries requiring formal irrigation and debridement (such as a fight bite or other suspected traumatic arthrotomy), those with an unstable joint, and those who have failed a complete trial of nonoperative management.

If necessary, smoking cessation, nutrition opti-mization, and blood glucose control are encour-aged in the perioperative period to provide an optimal environment for tendon healing. The will-ingness of the patient to comply with postopera-tive splinting and therapy protocols is also assessed. Although surgical treatment of extensor tendon injuries is not emergent, we prefer to oper-ate as soon as reasonably possible, generally within 1 week of the injury.

REPAIR TECHNIQUES

Our preference is to perform extensor mechanism repairs in a sterile operating suite either with local anesthesia and conscious sedation or regional anesthesia with an infraclavicular block. The patient is positioned supine with the arm on a hand table. We generally use a pneumatic tourni-quet. Although 4-0 FiberWire (Arthrex, Naples, FL) is our preferred suture because of its favorable biomechanical properties, any braided nonabsorb-able suture preferred by the surgeon can be used.[13] Larger 3-0 suture can be used in the more proximal portions of the tendon, such as zones VI to IX.

Zone I

Acute injuries

Most closed acute zone I (mallet finger) injuries can be treated nonoperatively. We prescribe full-time splinting for 8 weeks followed by night splinting for 4 weeks. We prefer a therapist-created custom mallet splint (**Fig. 1**), but similar splints that immobilize the DIP in full extension while allowing PIP motion are suitable. Careful instructions and patient compliance are critical to avoiding a subsequent extensor lag. Patients must be advised that they need to keep their DIP joint fully extended for 24 hours per day, 7 days per week. Patients should have more than 1 splint to facilitate hygiene and convenience. Physicians should also ensure that patients monitor their skin for breakdown or irritation.

Our preference is to surgically treat patients who have a zone I extensor tendon injury with an associated fracture (a bony mallet injury) that has more than 40% articular involvement or DIP subluxation/instability. We prefer the fluoroscopically aided extension block pinning technique first described by Ishiguro.[14–17] The DIP joint is flexed and a 0.89-mm or 1.14-mm (0.035-in″ or 0.045-in″) K-wire is inserted in a proximally directed orientation at approximately 45° into the distal aspect of the dorsal middle phalanx just dorsal to the fractured bony fragment of the distal phalanx. The DIP joint is then fully extended, allowing the pin to aid the reduction of the bony fragment. After ensuring that the DIP reduction is congruous, a retrograde K-wire is inserted longitudinally (centered on anteroposterior and lateral fluoroscopy images) across the DIP joint to immobilize the joint. If there is skin tenting, we make a small longitudinal incision with an 11-blade where the dorsal block pin will rest to minimize the risk of skin necrosis. Both wires are removed after 6 weeks if radiographic and clinical evidence of fracture healing are present (**Fig. 2**A, B).

For both nonoperative and surgical treatment, it is paramount to advise the patient to continue moving the PIP joint to avoid inadvertent joint stiffness. Patients should also be advised that a slight extensor lag may persist and full DIP joint flexion may not be possible despite seemingly successful treatment.

Chronic mallet injuries

For patients with chronic mallet finger injuries, a careful assessment is made of the patient's symptoms and functional deficits resulting from extensor lag. If the patient is asymptomatic and is without functional deficit, nonoperative management is continued with instructions for the patient to return for reevaluation if function becomes impaired. In patients with pain, degenerative arthritis of the DIP joint is excluded via clinical and radiographic examination. DIP arthrodesis is recommended if it is thought that the patient's symptoms are primarily attributable to degenerative joint disease.

For patients with a functional deficit or secondary swan neck deformity caused by a persistent extensor lag, we perform an imbrication of the terminal tendon to restore appropriate tension to the extensor mechanism. An H-type dorsal incision is made over the DIP joint and both the radial and ulnar aspects of the terminal tendon are exposed. A tenolysis is performed, with careful attention paid to ensuring that the palmar portion of the tendon is free of adhesions. The DIP joint is held in extension by placing a retrograde longitudinal K-wire with fluoroscopic assistance. The terminal tendon is transversely cut at the level of the DIP joint. The proximal part of the tendon is advanced distally until the appropriate tension has been restored in the extensor mechanism. A horizontal mattress suture is placed to secure the imbrication of the advanced proximal tendon to the distal terminal tendon (**Fig. 3**A, B). This technique allows a tendon-to-tendon healing environment. Although other investigators have described successful experiences with tenodermodesis and skin imbrication techniques, we prefer the advancement/imbrication technique because it preserves the thin surrounding soft tissue envelope.

Zones II and IV

Because the extensor tendons are broad and flat in these zones, we prefer to use the R-IHM suture configuration. The modified/augmented Becker (MGH) technique, modified Kessler, and modified Bunnell configurations are also commonly used by other surgeons. The R-IHM avoids the use of

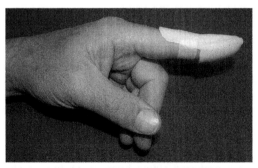

Fig. 1. Mallet finger splint, custom made with thermoplastic material by a certified hand therapist. It immobilizes the DIP joint but allows for motion at the PIP joint. (*Courtesy of* Hand Therapy, Hospital for Special Surgery.)

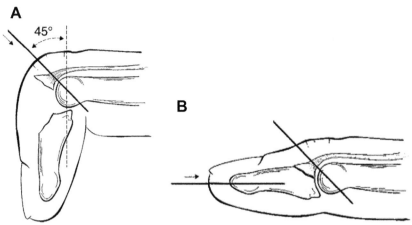

Fig. 2. (*A*) A 1.14-mm (0.045-in) K-wire is introduced under fluoroscopic guidance through the extensor tendon at a 45° angle into the distal portion of the middle phalanx with the DIP joint flexed. Arrow indicates direction of wire insertion. The distal phalanx is then extended and translated, compressing the fragment and acting as an extension block. Manipulation of the distal phalanx against the extension block K-wire is occasionally required to obtain an anatomic reduction. (*B*) A second K-wire is inserted longitudinally from distal to proximal across the DIP joint with the DIP joint extended. Arrow indicates direction of wire insertion. (*From* Hofmeister EP, Mazurek MT, Shin AY, et al. Extension block pinning for large mallet fractures. J Hand Surg Am 2003;28:455; with permission.)

core sutures in a flat tendon and is biomechanically strong enough to allow early motion. In these zones, we use a 4-0 braided nonabsorbable suture. A simple running suture is placed first, starting closest to the surgeon on the near end. On the far end of the tendon, an R-IHM suture is placed. Each step of the mattress configuration is locked by passing the suture needle underneath the preceding crossing suture. Once the last mattress suture is completed, the suture is tied on the near end (**Fig. 4**A, B). We also use the R-IHM suture configuration in purely tendinous zone I extensor tendon lacerations and in zone V extensor tendon injuries without sagittal band involvement. Our preference is to immobilize the DIP joint for 4 weeks, but early motion is allowed if deemed necessary because of concurrent injuries (such as a repaired flexor tendon that will be mobilized early).

Zone III: Central Slip

We initially treat acute closed central slip injuries nonoperatively by splinting the PIP in extension

with the DIP free for at least 4 weeks. For open injuries, the central slip is repaired with the R-IHM technique. If the remaining distal tendinous portion of the central slip is not robust enough for direct repair, a suture anchor can be applied to the middle phalanx to facilitate tendon-to-bone fixation. Injuries to the triangular ligament cause the lateral bands to migrate volarly, creating an acute boutonnière deformity. If this cannot be treated with primary repair, the triangular ligament's function can effectively be restored by suturing together the lateral bands distal to the PIP joint. The surgeon must be sure to avoid suturing the lateral bands together proximal to the PIP joint, because this would impede PIP joint flexion.

Zone V: Sagittal Band

Nonoperative management is initially attempted for acute closed sagittal band injuries. The finger is splinted with the MP joint in extension, leaving the IP joints free. This position, which can be accomplished with a sagittal band bridge splint or yoke splint, is held for 4 weeks (**Fig. 5**A, B).[18]

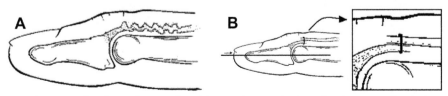

Fig. 3. (*A*) In a chronic mallet finger from a closed injury, the terminal tendon is present but lacks appropriate tension. (*B*) The DIP joint is extended and pinned using a 1.14-mm or 0.89-mm (0.045-in or 0.035-in) K-wire. Arrow indicates direction of wire insertion. The terminal tendon is transected and imbricated with 1 or 2 horizontal mattress sutures.

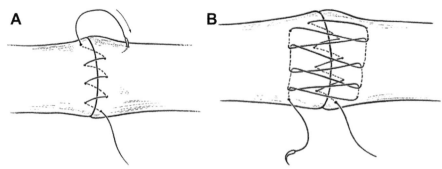

Fig. 4. (*A*) How to perform the new extensor tendon running interlocking horizontal mattress repair technique: begin the simple running suture at the near end. Arrow indicates orientation for suture to begin the horizontal mattress portion of the repair technique. (*B*) How to perform the new extensor tendon running interlocking horizontal mattress repair technique: run the interlocking horizontal mattress suture by starting at the far end. The suture needle passes underneath the prior crossing suture to lock each throw. Finish the suture and tie at the near end. (*From* Lee SK, Dubey A, Kim BH, et al. A biomechanical study of extensor tendon repair methods: introduction to the running-interlocking horizontal mattress extensor tendon repair technique. J Hand Surg Am 2010;35:21; with permission.)

For open injuries or those that have failed a complete trial of nonoperative management, direct repair of the sagittal bands is performed using a running simple suture or figure-of-eight suture configuration. In subacute or chronic injury, an attempt is also made to primarily repair the sagittal band. If the tissue quality is too poor to permit primary repair, we perform the extensor tendon centralization procedure described by Kang and Carlson.[19] A dorsal midline exposure is used to explore the sagittal band injury. Once the inability to repair local tissue has been confirmed, a local tendon graft (usually palmaris longus, EIP, or half of flexor carpi radialis) is harvested. A 1.6-mm drill bit is used to create a transverse

bone tunnel at the level of the metacarpal head-neck junction. The orientation of the drill can be adjusted at the surgeon's discretion depending on the position of extensor tendon subluxation. The extensor tendon is held in a centralized position and the graft is circumferentially woven through the transverse bony tunnel. The MP joint is passively ranged while ensuring that the extensor tendon remains in a central position. The graft pulley is sutured using 3-0 nonabsorbable braided suture. Fine adjustments in the pulley tension and overall orientation of the extensor tendon can be made by using additional sutures in remaining sagittal band tissue. The MP joint is mobilized early at approximately 1 week

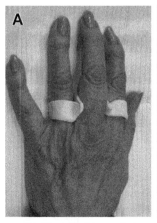
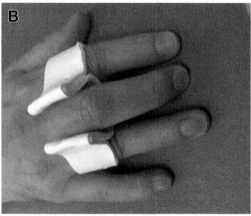

Fig. 5. (*A*) The sagittal band bridge splint used to treat a middle finger sagittal band injury. The splint provides 25° to 35° more extension of the MP joint compared with the adjacent digits. Note the centralized position of the EDC tendon of the middle finger. (*B*) Yoke splint for sagittal band ruptures. ([*A*] *From* Catalano III LW, Gupta S, Ragland III R, et al. Closed treatment of nonrheumatoid extensor tendon dislocations at the metacarpophalangeal joint. J Hand Surg Am 2006;31:243; with permission; and [*B*] *Courtesy of* Hand Therapy, Hospital for Special Surgery, New York, NY.)

postoperatively. As mentioned earlier, zone V extensor tendon lacerations without sagittal band involvement are treated similarly to zone II and IV injuries, with an R-IHM suture configuration and corresponding postoperative splinting and rehabilitation.

Zones VI, VII, VIII, and IX

Because these portions of the tendons are rounder, we prefer to use a modified Kessler technique with 3-0 nonabsorbable braided suture for acute repairs. This technique gives the benefit of the additional strength from the presence of the core sutures.

COMPLICATIONS

Static immobilization intended to protect freshly repaired extensor tendons can have the unintended result of joint stiffness.[20] In a series of 101 extensor tendon repairs that were followed by static splinting, loss of flexion was more problematic than extensor lag, particularly in zones III and IV.[20] Loss of flexion may have a greater effect on overall hand function, because grip strength and grasping ability are greatly affected.[21] Although dynamic motion protocols have decreased the frequency of postoperative joint stiffness, the surgeon should carefully balance the risks of joint stiffness and repair rupture during the initial postoperative period. However, the complications traditionally associated with flexor tendon repairs are not common. Rates of extensor tendon repair rupture historically have ranged from 0% to 8%, and rates of tenolysis after extensor tendon repair have ranged from 0% to 17%.[9,20,22–25]

CLINICAL OUTCOMES

In general, better outcomes are seen in proximal zones (zones V–VIII) than in distal zones (zones I–IV), largely because the tendon excursion is more forgiving proximally to adjustments in length and tension.[20] According to Miller's[26] scoring system, less than 50% of the patients in Newport's series who had zone I to IV injuries had good to excellent outcomes, whereas 63% to 83% of patients with zone V to VIII injuries had good to excellent outcomes. Modern suture techniques and rehabilitation protocols have improved outcomes, with good to excellent outcomes exceeding 90% for proximal injuries.[21,26,27] We have also seen favorable results with repair of distal extensor tendon lacerations. Patients often have full range of motion with an early range-of-motion postoperative protocol.

SUMMARY

Extensor tendon injuries occur frequently. An in-depth understanding of the intricate anatomy of the extensor mechanism is necessary to guide management. A trial of closed management is indicated for many extensor mechanism injuries and careful counseling is needed to ensure patient compliance and optimal outcomes. For bony mallet injuries that require surgery, we prefer extension block pinning. For distal extensor tendon lacerations in zones II to V, we prefer to use the R-IHM technique. It is important for the surgeon to avoid the unintended consequence of joint stiffness, which can occur from prolonged immobilization or inadvertent shortening of the extensor mechanism. In general, clinical outcomes have improved with modern repair techniques and rehabilitation programs.

REFERENCES

1. Clayton RA, Court-Brown CM. The epidemiology of musculoskeletal tendinous and ligamentous injuries. Injury 2008;39:1338–44.
2. O'Sullivan ME, Colville J. The economic impact of hand injuries. J Hand Surg Br 1993;18:395–8.
3. Gaul JS Jr. Identifiable costs and tangible benefits resulting from the treatment of acute injuries of the hand. J Hand Surg Am 1987;12:966–70.
4. Matzon JL, Bozentka DJ. Extensor tendon injuries. J Hand Surg Am 2010;35:854–61.
5. Stauch RJ. Extensor tendon injury. In: Wolfe SW, Hotchkiss RN, Pederson WC, et al, editors. Green's operative hand surgery. 6th edition. Philadelphia: Elsevier: Churchill Livingston; 2011. p. 159.
6. Shum C, Bruno RJ, Ristic S, et al. Examination of the anatomic relationship of the proximal germinal nail matrix to the extensor tendon insertion. J Hand Surg Am 2000;25:1114–7.
7. Kleinert HE, Verdan C. Report of the Committee on Tendon Injuries (International Federation of Societies for Surgery of the Hand). J Hand Surg Am 1983;8:794–8.
8. Doyle JR. Extensor tendons-acute injuries. In: Wolfe SW, Hotchkiss RN, Pederson WC, et al, editors. Green's operative hand surgery. 4th edition. New York: Elsevier: Churchill Livingston; 1999. p. 195.
9. Newport ML, Pollack GR, Williams CD. Biomechanical characteristics of suture techniques in extensor zone IV. J Hand Surg Am 1995;20:650–6.
10. Woo SH, Tsai TM, Kleinert HE, et al. A biomechanical comparison of four extensor tendon repair techniques in zone IV. Plast Reconstr Surg 2005;115:1674–81.
11. Howard RF, Ondrovic L, Greenwald DP. Biomechanical analysis of four-strand extensor tendon repair techniques. J Hand Surg Am 1997;22:838–42.

12. Lee SK, Dubey A, Kim BH, et al. A biomechanical study of extensor tendon repair methods: introduction to the running-interlocking horizontal mattress extensor tendon repair technique. J Hand Surg Am 2010;35:19–23.

13. Miller B, Dodds SD, deMars A, et al. Flexor tendon repairs: the impact of FiberWire on grasping and locking core sutures. J Hand Surg Am 2007;32:591–6.

14. Ishizuki M. Traumatic and spontaneous dislocation of extensor tendon of the long finger. J Hand Surg Am 1990;15:967–72.

15. Ishiguro T, Itoh Y, Yabe Y, et al. Extension block with Kirschner wire for fracture dislocation of the distal interphalangeal joint. Tech Hand Up Extrem Surg 1997;1:95–102.

16. Tetik C, Gudemez E. Modification of the extension block Kirschner wire technique for mallet fractures. Clin Orthop Relat Res 2002;404:284–90.

17. Hofmeister EP, Mazurek MT, Shin AY, et al. Extension block pinning for large mallet fractures. J Hand Surg Am 2003;28:453–9.

18. Catalano LW III, Gupta S, Ragland R III, et al. Closed treatment of nonrheumatoid extensor tendon dislocations at the metacarpophalangeal joint. J Hand Surg Am 2006;31:242–5.

19. Kang L, Carlson MG. Extensor tendon centralization at the metacarpophalangeal joint: surgical technique. J Hand Surg Am 2010;35: 1194–7.

20. Newport ML, Blair WF, Steyers CM Jr. Long-term results of extensor tendon repair. J Hand Surg Am 1990;15:961–6.

21. Newport ML, Tucker RL. New perspectives on extensor tendon repair and implications for rehabilitation. J Hand Ther 2005;18:175–81.

22. Browne EZ Jr, Ribik CA. Early dynamic splinting for extensor tendon injuries. J Hand Surg 1989; 14:72–6.

23. Chow JA, Dovelle S, Thomes LJ, et al. A comparison of results of extensor tendon repair followed by early controlled mobilisation versus static immobilisation. J Hand Surg Br 1989;14:18–20.

24. Crosby CA, Wehbé MA. Early protected motion after extensor tendon repair. J Hand Surg Am 1999;24: 1061–70.

25. Howell JW, Merritt WH, Robinson SJ. Immediate controlled active motion following zone 4–7 extensor tendon repair. J Hand Ther 2005;18:182–90.

26. Miller H. Repair of severed tendons of the hand and wrist. Surg Gynecol Obstet 1942;74:693–8.

27. Sameem M, Wood T, Ignacy T, et al. A systematic review of rehabilitation protocols after surgical repair of the extensor tendons in zones V-VIII of the hand. J Hand Ther 2011;24:365–72.

Diagnosis and Treatment of Finger Deformities Following Injuries to the Extensor Tendon Mechanism

Martin A. Posner, MD[a,b],*, Steven M. Green, MD[a,b]

KEYWORDS

- Extensor tendon anatomy • Boutonnière deformity • Intrinsic contracture and release

KEY POINTS

- Normal extension of the metacarpophalangeal, proximal interphalangeal, and distal interphalangeal joints depends on the coordinated action of the extrinsic extensor and intrinsic musculotendinous units as well as the static stabilizers.
- Careful physical examination is critical in the evaluation of injuries to the extensor mechanism.
- Treatment methods include immobilization and surgery.

The extensor digitorum communis (EDC) tendons to the 4 fingers, together with the extensor indicis proprius (EIP) to the index finger and the extensor digit quinti proprius (EDQP) to the little finger, begin in the forearm, course across the wrist and hand, and end at the metacarpophalangeal (MP) joints. They are independent tendons except on the dorsum of the hand where there are intertendinous connections referred to as juncturae tendinum. Distal to the MP joints the EDC, EIP, and EDQP tendons become the extrinsic component of the extensor tendon mechanism of each finger that also receives a component from the intrinsic muscles.

Injuries to the extensor tendons at the level of the MP joints and to the extensor tendon mechanisms in the fingers are common. These injuries and their treatment will be discussed at 4 anatomic sites: the MP joints, the dorsum of the proximal segments of the fingers, the dorsum of the proximal interphalangeal (PIP) joints, and the dorsum of the distal interphalangeal (DIP) joints.

MP JOINT

The extensor tendon in each finger is held in its normal midline dorsal position over the MP joint by radial and ulnar sagittal bands that insert into the sides of the volar plate, forming a closed cylindrical-like tube that surrounds the joint and the metacarpal head.[1] The radial sagittal bands are usually thinner and longer than the ulnar sagittal bands. The extensor tendons exert their force through both sagittal bands to the volar plates to form slinglike structures that extend the joints. Open injuries to the extensor tendons and sagittal bands are common, and should be repaired when lacerated. Repair of the extensor tendon restores MP joint extension, and repair of the sagittal band prevents displacement of the

a Division of Hand Surgery, Hospital for Joint Diseases, New York University, New York, NY, USA; b New York University School of Medicine, New York University, New York, NY, USA
* Corresponding author. New York University School of Medicine, New York University, 2 East 88 Street, New York, NY 10128.
E-mail address: mposner500@yahoo.com

Hand Clin 29 (2013) 269–281
http://dx.doi.org/10.1016/j.hcl.2013.03.003
0749-0712/13/$ – see front matter © 2013 Elsevier Inc. All rights reserved.

tendon to the opposite side. Even in the absence of injury to the extensor tendon itself, a sagittal band injury that is not repaired often results in an extension lag of the joint. Postoperatively, a volar splint is used to immobilize the wrist in moderate extension and the MP joints in approximately 30° of flexion. Immobilizing the MP joints of all 4 fingers rather than only the MP joint of the operated finger is preferred for 3 to 4 weeks to protect the surgical repair. A splint limited to the injured finger can then be used for an additional 2 weeks. Because the MP joints are immobilized in slight flexion, there is little risk that significant extension contractures will develop.

In some cases, an open injury to the dorsum of an MP joint is caused by a puncture wound from a tooth when an individual punches another in the mouth. These injuries are serious because of the high risk of infection, especially when treatment is delayed. Fist injuries are equivalent to human bites and require antibiotics as well as surgical exploration, irrigation, and debridement. The wound is left open, although when extensive, the skin edges can be loosely approximated with 1 or 2 sutures. The extensor tendon is rarely disrupted in these injuries, but there may be a defect in the radial or ulnar sagittal band.

Closed injuries to the dorsum of MP joints are far more common than open injuries, and the tendon dislocations that ensue are commonly classified into traumatic and spontaneous groups. Traumatic dislocations can follow a direct blow to the area, sudden forceful flexion of the joint, or a forceful torsion injury to the joint that frequently occurs in individuals who, while driving, are tightly gripping the steering wheel that suddenly spins in their hand. Patients in the spontaneous group of tendon dislocations may not be immediately aware of any injury and later recall that the problem followed what they thought was a seemingly trivial episode, such as opening a tight jar lid.

When discussing traumatic and spontaneous extensor tendon dislocations, it is important to understand the anatomy of their relationship to the sagittal bands. Each sagittal band consists of a superficial and deep layer. The superficial layers of the radial and ulnar sagittal bands form a continuous layer superficial to the tendon, whereas the thicker deep layers provide a groove for the tendon as it courses across the MP joint. There is no separation between superficial and deep layers, but there is a separation between the deep layer and the underlying joint capsule. The loose connective tissue in this interval can easily be dissected in order to mobilize the tendon. Traumatic extensor tendon dislocations are usually the result of tears in both superficial and deep layers of the radial sagittal band at a site several millimeters from the tendon. Spontaneous dislocations also result from tears in the sagittal band and, as with traumatic dislocations, it usually involves, the radial sagittal band. However, only the superficial layer is disrupted and at a site immediately adjacent to the tendon; the deep layer remains intact.[2]

Regardless of the cause, most closed traumatic and spontaneous extensor tendon dislocations involve the middle finger, followed in frequency by the ring finger.[3] The index and little fingers are not commonly involved, and the patterns of dislocations of the 2 tendons in each, the EDC and the proprius, can vary. In the index finger, both tendons can dislocate ulnarly when the tear is in the radial sagittal band, or the EDC can shift radially and the EIP ulnarly when the tear is between the tendons. In the little finger, dislocations of the EDC and EDQP can follow similar patterns. However, the little finger differs from the index finger in that the EDC is absent in most individuals and is replaced by a junctura tendinum that attaches the ring finger EDC to the extensor aponeurosis of the little finger just proximal to the MP joint.[4]

The treatment of closed traumatic and spontaneous tendon dislocation injuries depends on their severity and the temporal interval between injury and diagnosis. In many cases, the tendon does not actually dislocate into the groove between the metacarpal heads but rather shifts slightly from its normal midline position over the MP joint, usually in an ulnar direction; the tendon subluxates rather than dislocates. When the subluxation is mild and not accompanied by any snap of the tendon with MP flexion, there is rarely a disability and treatment is not required. However, a subluxated or dislocated tendon that snaps with joint flexion usually requires treatment. For the acute problem, and generally this is considered to be within 2 weeks of the injury, the injured finger is immobilized in sufficient MP extension to permit the tendon to resume its normal midline position.[5] This position is easily determined by passively extending the MP joint and noting the position where the extensor tendon spontaneously relocates to its normal position. Generally, it is approximately 20° of flexion, and this is the position that the joint is immobilized rather than in full extension, which is more likely to result in an extension contracture. The most comfortable and effective splint is palm based and fabricated by a hand therapist from a thermoplastic material that immobilizes only the MP joint (**Fig. 1**). The splint should not interfere with interphalangeal joint motions and is worn for 4 to 5 weeks. Patients can remove it to bathe provided they do not attempt to flex the MP joint.

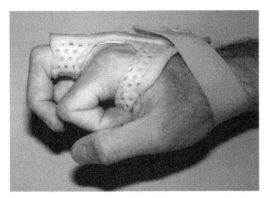

Fig. 1. Effective treatment of the acute or subacute extensor tendon dislocation is achieved with a static palm-based splint that immobilizes the MP joint in slight flexion and does not interfere with motions of the interphalangeal joints.

For chronic injuries of more than 2 weeks duration, surgery is usually necessary unless the extensor tendon still spontaneously shifts back to its normal midline position with MP extension. In such cases, a splint is used. However, splint immobilization is not as effective for chronic injuries as it is for acute injuries, and patients should be informed that they could require later surgery. When surgery is performed, all that is necessary, in most cases, is to mobilize the extensor tendon, restore it to its midline position over the MP joint, and repair the tear in the radial sagittal band to maintain the tendon in its correct position. In some chronic cases, the fibers of the intact ulnar sagittal band have contracted and they must be divided via a longitudinal incision to permit relocation of the extensor tendon. It may also be necessary to imbricate the radial sagittal fibers to stabilize the tendon after it is restored to its proper position (**Fig. 2**). When imbrication of the radial sagittal band is not feasible because the tissues are too attenuated, a different procedure is

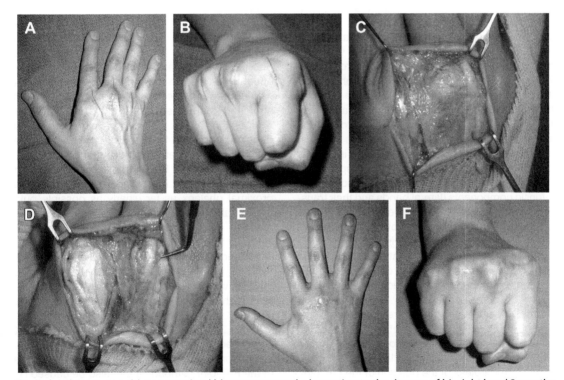

Fig. 2. (*A*, *B*) A 25-year-old man sustained blunt trauma and a laceration to the dorsum of his right hand 2 months earlier. The laceration was sutured in a local emergency department; following removal of the sutures 1 week later, he received no further medical care. He noted that the index and middle fingers were deviated, and examination showed that the extensor tendons were ulnarly subluxated. (*C*) At surgery, the radial sagittal fibers in both fingers were attenuated, more in the middle finger than the index finger, and the ulnar sagittal fibers in both fingers had undergone secondary contractures. (*D*) To relocate the extensor tendons, it was necessary to divide the ulnar sagittal fibers in both fingers (probe on cut fibers in middle finger) and reef the radial sagittal fibers. (*E*, *F*) Postoperatively, the extensor tendons were restored to their normal midline positions over the MP joints, and digital mobility was complete.

required to stabilize the tendon in its normal position. A variety of operative techniques have been described that generally report favorable results.[6] Most techniques involve using a strip of the extensor tendon, either from its radial or ulnar side, that is looped around the lumbrical or the radial collateral ligament or is passed through the deep transverse metacarpal ligament.[7-10] Regardless of the technique, postoperative immobilization is similar to that used for acute closed injuries; the MP joints of all fingers are immobilized as well as the wrist that is positioned in moderate extension for the first 3 to 4 weeks followed by a palm-based splint confined to the injured finger for another 2 weeks.

DORSUM OF PROXIMAL SEGMENT

The distal extension of the extrinsic EDC in the finger is the central tendon (often referred to as the central slip) that courses over the proximal phalanx and inserts into the base of the middle phalanx. Attached to the radial and ulnar sides of the central tendon are transverse and oblique fibers from the lateral bands that arise from the intrinsic muscles. The extrinsic central tendon and the intrinsic lateral bands, together with their transverse and oblique fibers, cover approximately 75% of the circumference of a proximal phalanx on its dorsal, radial, and ulnar surfaces. The only surface of the phalanx not covered is the volar surface that is the site of attachment for the flexor tendon sheath and where the flexor superficialis and profundus tendons course distally to their insertions on the middle and distal phalanges, respectively. Scarring of the extrinsic (central tendon) and intrinsic components (lateral bands and their transverse and oblique fibers) of the extensor tendon mechanism are common following fractures of the proximal phalanx or following less severe injuries that result in swelling that leads to scarring and adhesions. In most cases, either the extrinsic or intrinsic component is scarred to the underlying bone; in some cases both components are scarred. Identifying the scarred component is determined by clinical examination. With scarring of the extrinsic tendon component, there is an extension contracture of the PIP joint that is unchanged regardless of the position of the MP joint. With scarring of the intrinsic tendon component to the radial and/or ulnar side of the phalanx the clinical examination can be identical with respect to the extension contracture of the PIP joint. However, most cases of scarring of the intrinsic component are more proximal in the interossei muscles themselves, which is evident by performing the Bunnell test for intrinsic tightness.

The Bunnell test is a completely passive test that has 2 parts and is performed with the patient's hand totally relaxed. In part one, the examiner positions the MP joint in maximum extension that is usually hyperextension that results in the intrinsics to the finger being stretched because they are volar to the axis of MP motions. The examiner then attempts to passively flex the PIP joint and determines if there is any limitation and the degree of that limitation. When passive PIP flexion is complete with the MP joint maximally extended, the intrinsics are normal and are not contracted. However, when passive PIP flexion is limited, part two of the test is performed to determine if the limitation in passive PIP flexion is caused by the contracture of the joint capsule. The examiner now positions the MP joint in full flexion, which relaxes the intrinsics, and again attempts to passively flex the PIP joint. When passive PIP flexion is limited with MP hyperextension but not with MP flexion, there are contractures of the intrinsics and not the joint capsule. Often, the intrinsic on one side of a finger is more contracted than the intrinsic on the opposite side, which can be determined by not only hyperextending the MP joint but also pushing the proximal phalanx in its hyperextended position as far ulnarly as possible and then as far radially as possible. The effect when pushing the phalanx ulnarly is that the intrinsic on the radial side of the finger is stretched more than the intrinsic on the ulnar side of the finger. Pushing the phalanx radially does the opposite; the intrinsic on the ulnar side of the finger is stretched more than the intrinsic on the radial side. For example, hyperextending the MP joint of an index finger and pushing the proximal phalanx as far ulnarly as possible puts the radial intrinsic, the first dorsal interosseous muscle, under greater stretch than the ulnar intrinsic, the first volar interosseous muscle. Hyperextending the MP joint and pushing it as far radial as possible has the opposite effect, it puts the first volar interosseous muscle under greater stretch than the first dorsal interosseous muscle (**Fig. 3**).

When PIP flexion is limited with the MP joint positioned in hyperextension and also in flexion, the reason is almost always a capsular contracture of the PIP joint, although it can also be caused by isolated scarring of the central tendon to the dorsum of the proximal phalanx. Differentiating between the two diagnoses may not be possible on a clinical examination but can usually be anticipated when considering the nature of the injury. For example, a patient who sustained a fracture of the proximal phalanx that healed with bony callus under the central tendon is more likely to

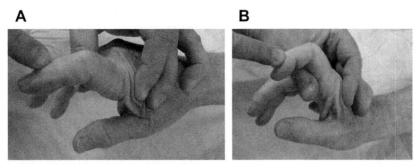

Fig. 3. (*A*) The MP joint when hyperextended and deviated radially results in tension on the first volar interosseous that is tight. (*B*) Deviating the hyperextended MP joint ulnarly showed that there was no tightness of the first dorsal interosseous muscle.

have scarring of the central tendon than having a contracture of the PIP joint capsule, although a capsular contracture can develop as a secondary problem in chronic cases. At surgery, attention is first directed to lysing the adhesions of the central tendon to the underlying proximal phalanx. A PIP capsulectomy is necessary when PIP passive flexion remains limited after the tenolysis is completed (**Fig. 4**). An extension contracture of a PIP joint also does not exclude the possibility that there are also intrinsic contractures because

both problems frequently coexist. It is, therefore, important to perform the Bunnell test at surgery following a PIP joint capsulectomy to determine if there are concomitant intrinsic contractures. When present, intrinsic releases are necessary.

There are 2 types of intrinsic releases that are classified according to the site where they are performed. When performed proximal to the MP joint, they are referred to as *proximal intrinsic releases* and when performed distal to the MP joint, *distal intrinsic releases* (**Fig. 5**). The indication to perform

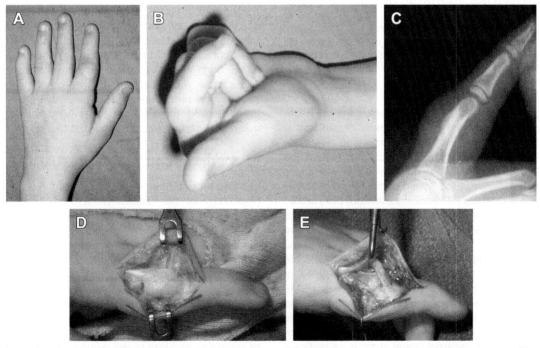

Fig. 4. (*A, B*) A 6-year-old child had sustained a crush-type injury to the dorsum of the proximal segment of her left index finger several months earlier. The child was unable to actively flex the PIP joint, and there was a block to passive flexion. (*C*) A lateral radiograph showed periosteal bone formation beneath the central tendon. (*D*) At surgery, the central tendon was scarred to the phalanx. (*E*) A tenolysis was performed, and the child regained almost complete finger mobility.

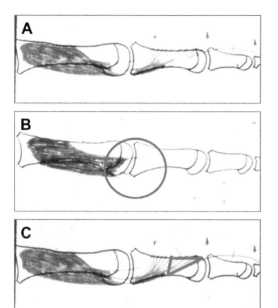

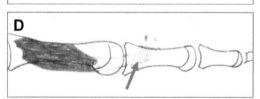

Fig. 5. (*A*) A lateral band and its transverse and oblique fibers that attach to the central extensor tendon. (*B*) A proximal intrinsic release. (*C*) The triangle of tissue consisting of the lateral band and its oblique fibers that are excised in a distal intrinsic release. (*D*) The results of a distal intrinsic release that preserves the transverse fibers arising from the lateral band.

one type of intrinsic release versus the other depends on the site of the contracture and that is determined by a clinical examination. Because the intrinsics flex the MP joints and extend the PIP joints, active and passive motions of these joints are evaluated. When active MP joint extension and active PIP flexion are limited, the intrinsic contracture is proximal to the MP joint, and it is this area that the intrinsics must be released, both at their insertions into the proximal phalanx and the lateral bands. Proximal intrinsic contractures are common in patients with inflammatory types of arthritis, such as rheumatoid arthritis, whose MP joints are often volarly subluxated. Arthroplasties of the MP joints with the insertion of silicone implants are proximal releases because with excision of the metacarpal heads, there is a significant decrease in the distances between the origins and insertions of the intrinsic muscles.

Most patients with intrinsic contractures have no problems with MP joint motions, only PIP joint

motions. Because their MP motions are normal, the components of the intrinsics that affect that joint, namely, the insertions of the intrinsic muscles on the bases of the proximal phalanges and the transverse fibers that extend from the lateral bands to the central tendon and assist in MP flexion, need not be disturbed. These patients do not need proximal intrinsic releases but rather distal intrinsic releases. For each involved finger, it consists of excision of the triangle of tissue composing one or both lateral bands and their oblique fibers; the transverse fibers are preserved. A distal intrinsic release is performed through a longitudinal incision on the dorsum of the proximal segment of the finger. Visualizing the lateral band with its transverse and oblique fibers is not difficult and is facilitated by deviating the finger in the opposite direction that puts the fibers under stretch (**Fig. 6**). The Bunnell test that was performed preoperatively is repeated at surgery to determine if the intrinsic on one side of the finger is more contracted than the intrinsic on the other side of the finger. When they are contracted on both sides and the contractures are of equal severity, it is dealer's choice in deciding which intrinsic lateral band and oblique fibers are excised first. In those cases when there is deviation of the MP joint to one side, it is preferable to first excise the intrinsic on that side because it is usually tighter than the intrinsic on the opposite side. In some cases, intrinsic tightness is not relieved following excision of one lateral band and its oblique fibers, and it is then necessary to excise the lateral band and oblique fibers on the other side of the finger. A distal intrinsic release is not a difficult surgical procedure, and its beneficial effects in eliminating the contracture are immediately evident by performing a Bunnell test.

PIP JOINT: THE BOUTONNIÈRE DEFORMITY

In 1930, Mason[11] succinctly explained the pathophysiology of the deformity: "It is the middle portion of the dorsal aponeurosis which ruptures, the two lateral slips now loosen from their attachment about the joint slip palmarward, and the joint comes to lie between them as in a 'buttonhole'."[11]

The deformity in English-speaking countries is referred to by the French word for buttonhole, that is, *boutonnière*; in French-speaking countries, it has been curiously Anglicized and is referred to as *deformitè buttonhole*. The deformity consists of weakness and loss of extension of the PIP joint and hyperextension and diminished active and passive flexion of the DIP joint (**Fig. 7**). It begins with disruption of the central tendon (**Fig. 8**) that is often caused by sudden forced flexion of a PIP

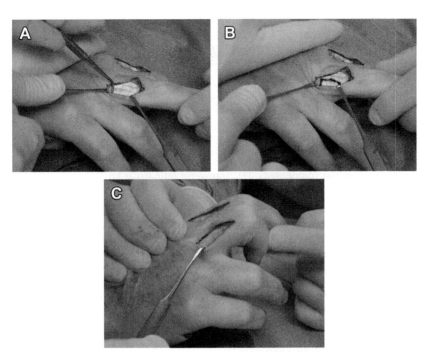

Fig. 6. (*A*) Surgical sequence for a distal intrinsic release of the ulnar intrinsic (third dorsal interosseous) in a middle finger following similar surgery for the index finger. The operative incision is longitudinal over the middle of the proximal finger segment that provides excellent visualization of the central tendon, the ulnar lateral band, and its transverse and oblique fibers. (*B*) The triangle of tissue consisting of the lateral band and the oblique fibers is outlined before excision. (*C*) Following excision of the triangle of tissue, a Bunnell test is performed to insure that the preoperative intrinsic contracture was eliminated.

joint that is actively being extended, resulting in an eccentric load on the finger. The central tendon can also be injured by an open injury, such as a laceration (**Fig. 9**), follow an infection, chemical or thermal injury, or result from an inflammatory type of arthritis (**Fig. 10**). In some cases, the central tendon disruption is accompanied by volar dislocation of the PIP joint (**Fig. 11**), or (rarely) the tendon avulses with a fragment from the dorsal base of the middle phalanx. The triangular ligament that connects the 2 lateral bands may be

initially injured together with the central tendon or it subsequently becomes stretched, permitting the lateral bands to shift volar to the axis of the PIP joint. Contractures of the oblique retinacular ligament, the volar plate of the PIP joint, and the collateral ligaments of the DIP joint then ensue (**Figs. 12** and **13**).

Boutonnière deformities have been classified into 5 stages.[12,13]

Stage 1: Active extension of the PIP joint may be weak, and the joint may be in a slightly flexed position; but active extension is still possible via the lateral bands that essentially remain in their normal anatomic positions.

Stage 2: The triangular ligament has attenuated, and there is a volar shift of both lateral bands volar to the axis of joint motions. Active extension of the PIP joint is now seriously affected.

Stage 3: There is progressive hyperextension of the DIP joint because the extension force of the intrinsic muscles is exclusively to that joint. Active and passive flexion of the DIP joint is also limited because of the contracture of the oblique retinacular ligaments.

Fig. 7. Boutonnière deformity with flexion of the PIP joint and hyperextension of the DIP joint.

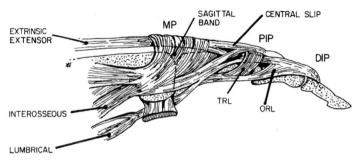

Fig. 8. Normal static and dynamic components. TRL, transverse retinacular lig; OBL, oblique retinacular lig.

Stage 4: There is a fixed flexion contracture of the PIP joint because of the contracture of the volar plate.

Stage 5: The boutonnière deformity is associated with articular degeneration of the PIP joint.

Elson described a diagnostic clinical examination technique to evaluate the integrity of the central slip by positioning the PIP in 90° of flexion and comparing the resting position of the DIP joint with the same joint in the contralateral uninjured digit.[14] He then asked the patient to actively extend the PIP joint of the injured finger against resistance; he noted that when the central tendon was disrupted, the active PIP joint extension was weak. The DIP joint also hyperextended, and passive flexion was restricted. Boyes[15] noted that with central tendon ruptures, active flexion of the DIP joint was limited when the PIP joint was passively positioned in full extension. Rubin[16] evaluated the diagnostic effectiveness of the Elson and Boyes methods, as well as other methods, using cadaver digits and concluded that the Elson test was the most effective diagnostic test.[16–19]

Treatment of a boutonnière deformity depends on its stage. For the acute injury (within the first 2 weeks), immobilization of the proximal interphalangeal joint in full extension for 4 to 5 weeks using a static splint that permits active and passive flexion of the DIP joint is usually effective (**Fig. 14**). Surgery is recommended only for an acute laceration of the central tendon or for a closed injury when the tendon avulses with a fragment from the dorsal base of the middle phalanx.

Subacute injuries (2–8 weeks) may present with either supple or stiff joints. When the PIP is supple and can be passively extended and there is no laceration or fracture, extension splinting, as for the acute injury, is the treatment of choice. However, when the injury is caused by a laceration or there is a displaced fracture fragment, surgery is necessary. Often, there are early flexion contractures in subacute injuries that are not yet fixed and respond to dynamic and/or static progressive extension splints. Frequently, sufficient joint motions can be restored with these splints that surgery can be avoided.

The treatment of the chronic injury (more than 8 weeks) is significantly more complicated because disruption of the central tendon is no longer an isolated problem. The triangular ligament has become attenuated, and the lateral bands have displaced volar to the axis of the PIP joint where they usually become fixed because of secondary contractures of the transverse retinacular ligaments. The oblique retinacular ligaments usually also contract together with the volar plate of the PIP joint and the collateral ligaments of the DIP joint. In those patients whose interphalangeal joints remain supple, an anatomic repair is recommended to restore active PIP joint extension. The operation is performed through a curved dorsal skin incision with its apex midaxial on either the

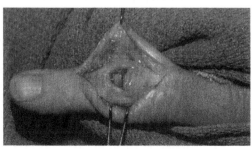

Fig. 9. Laceration of the central tendon.

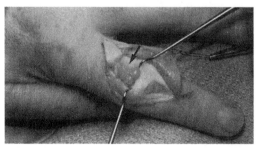

Fig. 10. Rheumatoid pannus (*arrow*) seen after reflection of the central slip.

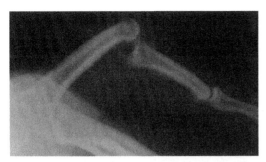

Fig. 11. Volar PIP joint dislocation.

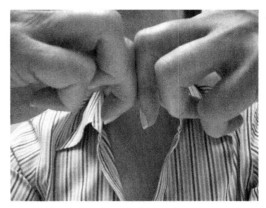

Fig. 13. Elson test. Note exaggerated DIP extension of the injured right middle finger.

radial or ulnar side of the finger. Elevation of the skin flap permits excellent visualization of the central slip that is usually retracted, the subluxated radial and ulnar lateral bands, and the contracted transverse retinacular ligaments. Incisions are made on the volar margins of both lateral bands, releasing them from their connections to the transverse retinacular ligaments. This release permits the lateral bands to be shifted back to their normal anatomic positions dorsal to the axis of PIP joint motions. The scarred and attenuated triangular ligament is excised, and the lateral bands are suture together at that site with 2 or 3 sutures of a fine grade (4–0 or 5–0). It is important not to insert any sutures proximal to the PIP joint that would likely result in an extension contracture. If possible, the central tendon and redundant scar tissue are elevated off the middle phalanx, and the central tendon is reattached into the middle phalanx using a small bone anchor (**Fig. 15**). In some cases, the central tendon has retracted and it may not be possible to reattach it. The PIP joint is temporarily stabilized with a Kirschner wire to facilitate early mobilization of the DIP joint. The wire is removed in 4 to 6 weeks, when active PIP exercises are encouraged.

When the integrity of the central tendon has been severely compromised, a variety of operative procedures have been described to restore its function. Mattev[20] recommended cutting one lateral band at the distal extent of the triangular ligament and the other lateral band at the base of the middle phalanx. The shorter of the two lateral bands was then passed through the proximal portion of the central slip and inserted into the dorsal base of the middle phalanx. The longer lateral band that had been cut at the triangular ligament was then sutured to the distal portion of the contralateral lateral band, thus creating an elongated lateral band. Littler and Eaton[21] suggested a reconstruction that involved separating the interosseous tendons from the lumbrical tendon and from the oblique retinacular ligament. The interosseous tendons are then rolled dorsally and sutured together at the level of the middle phalanx. Distal joint extension is preserved through the oblique retinacular ligament. Hellman and later Aiche and colleagues[22,23] described a technique that involved splitting the lateral bands longitudinally and approximating the medial halves together to reconstruct the central tendon. When local tendon tissue is insufficient, a free tendon graft is usually required. The midportion of the graft is attached to the dorsal base of the middle phalanx, and the ends are crossed dorsally and sutured into the lateral bands proximal to the PIP joint.[24,25] An alternative technique would be a transfer of a slip of the flexor digitorum superficialis tendon to a lateral band (**Fig. 16**).

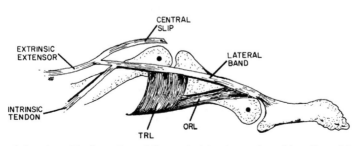

Fig. 12. Boutonnière deformity with disruption of the central tendon, volar subluxation of the lateral bands, and contractures of the transverse (TRL) and oblique retinacular ligaments (OBL).

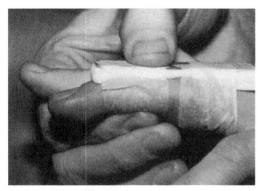

Fig. 14. A splint that immobilizes the PIP in full extension and permits DIP flexion.

For patients who present with an unacceptable fixed flexion contracture of the PIP joint that has not responded to dynamic and/or static progressive splinting, correction of the joint contracture is the first requirement. Stretching the volar plate can be accomplished using an external fixator or surgically via a capsulectomy involving the volar plate and accessory collateral ligaments and, in some cases, the volar portions of the collateral ligaments. The transverse retinacular ligaments are sectioned to mobilize the lateral bands. Correction of the PIP flexion contracture alone is sometimes sufficient. However, if the joint can made supple, a tendon reconstruction is performed for those patients unable to regain adequate active PIP extension.

For many patients, their main functional complaint is the hyperextension deformity of the DIP joint rather than the deficit in active PIP

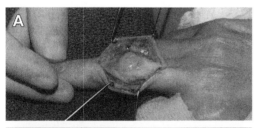

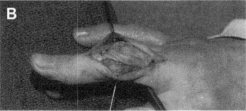

Fig. 15. (*A*) Intense scarring of central tendon and lateral bands. (*B*) Anatomic repair of central tendon, and mobilization and imbrication of lateral bands. (Note: sutures in the lateral bands are distal to PIP joint).

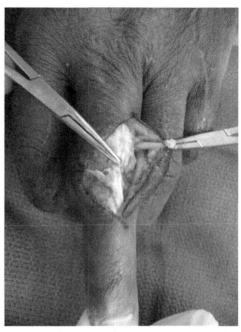

Fig. 16. Transfer of the flexor digitorum superficialis (FDS) to one lateral band.

extension. In such cases, a tenotomy of the lateral bands distal to the insertion of the central slip improves the hyperextension deformity of the DIP joint. A severe mallet deformity does not occur because the oblique retinacular ligament remains intact. The tenotomy, first described by Fowler[25] and later reported by others, diminishes the flexion position of the PIP joint because it increases tension of the lateral bands that is transmitted to the damaged central tendon (**Fig. 17**).[25–27]

When a chronic boutonnière deformity is associated with arthritis of the proximal interphalangeal joint that is painful, an arthrodesis is an effective procedure to relieve pain and position the joint in a functional position. In selected patients who want to maintain active joint motions and whose extensor tendon mechanism is amenable to reconstruction, an implant arthroplasty can be considered. The procedure requires mobilization of what remains of the central tendon, mobilization of the lateral bands, insertion of the implant, followed by a tendon reconstruction, as previously described.

DIP JOINT

Extensor tendon injuries at the DIP joint are among the most frequent injuries that affect the hand. The injury usually results from a sudden flexion force applied to an extended finger that disrupts either partially or completely the conjoined lateral bands at or near their insertion into

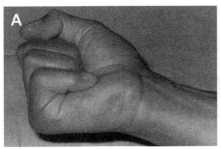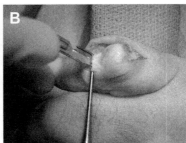

Fig. 17. (*A*) Loss of DIP flexion that affected patient's ability to forcefully grip a hammer. (*B*) Extensor tenotomy performed at level of the probe distal to the triangular ligament.

the base of the distal phalanx. There is a loss of active extension of the DIP joint that varies according to the degree of tendon injury that may simply be attenuated or completely disrupted. In most cases, there is not a complete disruption, and the loss of extension is in the 30° to 40° range. The flexed position of the DIP joint is commonly referred to as a *mallet finger* or *baseball finger*, although *drop finger* or *droop finger* are more accurate descriptions.[28] These injuries are often associated with degenerative DIP joint arthritis that, together with the avascular zone in the tendon that is located approximately 1.0 to 1.5 cm from its insertion where it passes over the head of the middle phalanx, compromises its integrity and makes it susceptible to rupture with even minor trauma, especially in the elderly.[29] In some cases, the tendon avulses with a bone fragment from the dorsal base of the distal phalanx. A lateral radiograph should, therefore, always be taken.

Numerous articles have appeared in the medical literature regarding the treatment of terminal extensor tendon injuries, and the vast majority recommend nonoperative measures. Splinting should be confined to the DIP joint and should not interfere with motions of the PIP joint. A dorsal splint is preferable to a volar splint because it is less likely to interfere with prehensile activities (**Fig. 18**). The splint should obviously be comfortable because it must be maintained for approximately 6 weeks. Patients must never permit the DIP joint to flex during this period, even for a split second; joint extension must be maintained 24 hours a day, 7 days a week. Patients can be taught to remove the splint each day to clean the dorsal skin without permitting the DIP joint to flex. This is easier with a dorsal splint than a volar splint, although it can also be accomplished with a well-fabricated volar splint (**Fig. 19**).

Splinting is also the preferred treatment of the closed extensor tendon injury that occurs with an

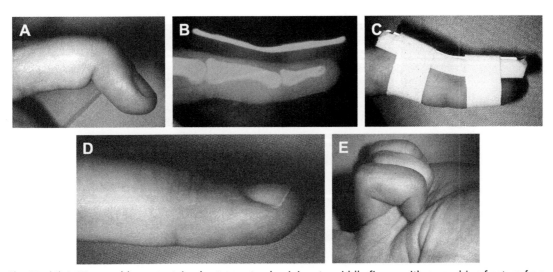

Fig. 18. (*A*) A 65-year-old man sustained extensor tendon injury to middle finger with no avulsion fracture fragment. (*B, C*) A lateral radiograph was negative, and an extension splint was applied to the dorsum of the DIP joint. (*D, E*) Following splinting for 8 weeks, complete extension restored with no loss of flexion.

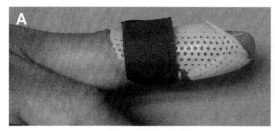
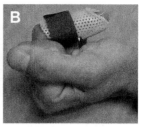

Fig. 19. (*A, B*) Another type of DIP extension splint fabricated by a hand therapist that permits normal motions of the PIP joint.

avulsion fracture, provided the joint is not volarly subluxated. However, extension splinting must be continued longer than for the nonavulsion injury until there is radiographic evidence of bone healing (**Fig. 20**). The avulsed fragment usually heals with a permanent bony prominence at the dorsal base of the distal phalanx. Although it has no functional significance, patients should still be alerted that it is likely to occur.

The only indication for operative treatment is when the avulsion fracture fragment is large and there is volar subluxation of the remaining portion of the bone resulting in articular incongruity. In those cases, the least invasive procedure that reduces the subluxated phalanx and stabilizing it is preferred. This procedure can usually be achieved with a Kirschner wire that is drilled percutaneously across the joint into the middle phalanx.

Individuals with a chronic drop finger often seek medical attention only because they do not like the aesthetic appearance of their finger. They often refer to it as disfiguring when actually the flexed position of the DIP joint is far more obvious to

them than to others because when hands are relaxed, fingers are also relaxed and slightly flexed; the DIP joints are never fully extended. The treatment of a chronic injury is necessary only when the DIP joint is in such severe flexion (generally that is at least 60°) that patients report a significant disability with important daily activities, such as typing at a computer or playing a musical instrument. In the absence of a significant disability, surgery should be avoided. Patients will generally accept that advice when they are told that an operation will not restore normal mobility; may result in an extension contracture that could compromise grasp; and, probably what is the most important, that it will result in scarring over the dorsum of the joint that will be far more noticeable than the current flexed position of the joint.

In the rare case of a chronic drop finger that is disabling, surgery is warranted. It is also warranted when there is hyperextension of the PIP joint that often occurs in patients with normal joint laxity. With disruption or attenuation of the terminal tendon, the lateral bands retract proximally and

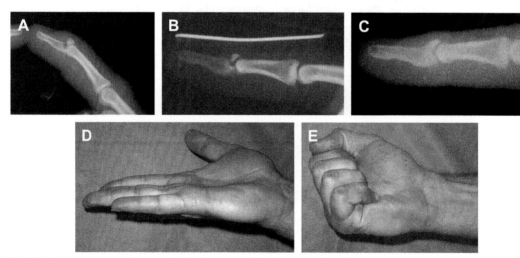

Fig. 20. Extensor tendon injury to index fingers with a large avulsion fragment but with no subluxation of the joint (*A, B*). A dorsal extension splint was used until there was bone healing that took 10 weeks (*C*). There was a slight bony prominence at the dorsum of the distal phalanx, and essentially full mobility was restored (*D, E*).

exert a greater extension force on the lax PIP joint that becomes hyperextended. The finger assumes a swan-neck appearance, with the hyperextended PIP joint resembling the neck of a swan and the flexed DIP joint resembling its head. This appearance is commonly seen in patients with rheumatoid arthritis and is usually caused by intrinsic contractures, whereas in patients with a chronic drop finger, the deformity is caused by an imbalance of extension forces at the PIP joint that ensues after the extension force at the DIP joint has been damaged. As with surgery for the chronic drop finger without PIP hyperextension, the surgery for the finger with PIP hyperextension is the same. The scarred segment of extensor tendon over the DIP joint is excised; by closing the gap, the imbalance of extension forces at the PIP joint is corrected, and a greater extension force to the DIP joint is restored.

SUMMARY

Injuries to the finger extensor apparatus are very common and may produce chronic deformity and loss of function. The diagnosis is contingent on an understanding of the complex anatomy of this region as well as the ability to perform a careful physical examination. Immobilization is usually the most effective treatment of acute problems. Surgery is often necessary for chronic conditions, but the results are much less predictably corrective.

REFERENCES

1. Young CM, Rayan GM. The sagittal band: anatomic and biomechanical study. J Hand Surg Am 2000;25: 1107–13.
2. Ishizuki M. Traumatic and spontaneous dislocations of extensor tendons of the long finger. J Hand Surg Am 1990;15:967–72.
3. Koniuch MP, Peimer CA, Van Gorder T, et al. Closed crush injury of the metacarpophalangeal joint. J Hand Surg Am 1987;12:750–7.
4. Schenck RR. Variations of the extensor tendons of the fingers: surgical significance. J Bone Joint Surg Am 1964;46:103–10.
5. Inoue G, Tamura Y. Dislocation of the extensor tendons over the metacarpophalangeal joints. J Hand Surg Am 1996;21:464–9.
6. Vaccaro AR, Kupcha P, Schneider LH. The operative repair of chronic non-traumatic extensor tendon subluxations in the hand. Hand Clin 1995;11:431–40.
7. McCoy FJ, Winsky AJ. Lumbrical loop operation luxation of the extensor tendons of the hand. Plast Reconstr Surg 1969;44:142–6.
8. Kilgore ES, Graham WP, Newmeyer WL, et al. Correction of ulnar subluxation of the extensor communis. Hand 1975;7:272–4.
9. Carroll C, Moore R, Weiland AJ. Post-traumatic ulnar subluxations of the extensor tendons: a reconstructive technique. J Hand Surg Am 1987;12:227–31.
10. Watson HK, Weinsweig J, Guidera PM. Sagittal band reconstruction. J Hand Surg Am 1997;22:452–6.
11. Mason ML. Rupture of tendons of the hand. Surg Gynecol Obstet 1930;50:611.
12. Zancolli E. Structural and dynamic basis of hand surgery. Philadelphia: JB Lippincott; 1968. p. 105.
13. Coons MS, Green SM. Boutonniere deformity. Hand Clin 1995;11:387–402.
14. Elson RA. Rupture of the central slip of the extensor hood of the finger. J Bone Joint Surg Br 1986;68: 229–31.
15. Boyes JH. Bunnel's surgery of the hand. 5th edition. Philadelphia: JB Lippincott; 1970. p. 393.
16. Rubin L, Bozentha DJ, Bora FW. Diagnosis of closed central slip injuries. J Hand Surg Br 1996;21:614–6.
17. Carducci T. Potential boutonnière deformity: its recognition and treatment. Orthop Rev 1981;10:121–3.
18. Lovett WL, McCalla MA. Management and rehabilitation of extensor injuries. Orthop Clin North Am 1983;14:811–26.
19. Smith PJ, Ross RA. The central slip tenodesis test for early diagnosis of potential boutonniere deformities. J Hand Surg Br 1994;19:88–90.
20. Matev I. Transposition of the lateral slips of the aponeurosis in treatment of long standing boutonniere deformity of the fingers. Br J Plast Surg 1964; 17:281–6.
21. Littler JW, Eaton RG. Redistribution of forces in the correction of the boutonnière deformity. J Bone Joint Surg Am 1967;49:1267–74.
22. Hellman K. Die wiederherstellung der strecksehen im bereich der fingermittelgelenke. Langebbecks Arch Surg 1964;309:36.
23. Aiche A, Barsky AJ, Weiner DL. Prevention of boutonnière deformity. Plast Reconstr Surg 1970;46:164–7.
24. Nichols HM. Repair of the extensor tendon insertions of the fingers. J Bone Joint Surg Am 1951; 33:836–41.
25. Fowler SB. The management of tendon injuries. J Bone Joint Surg Am 1959;41:579–80.
26. Dolphin JA. Extensor tenotomy for chronic boutonnière deformity of the finger. J Bone Joint Surg Am 1965;47:161–4.
27. Meadows SE, Schneider LH, Sherwyn JH. Treatment of the chronic boutonnière deformity by extensor tenotomy. Hand Clin 1995;11:441–7.
28. Abouna JM, Brown H. The treatment of mallet finger. Br J Surg 1968;55:653–66.
29. Warren RA, Kay NR, Norris SH. The microvascular anatomy of the distal extensor tendon. J Hand Surg Br 1988;13:161–3.

Complex Flexor and Extensor Tendon Injuries

Matthew J. Carty, MD[a],*, Philip E. Blazar, MD[b]

KEYWORDS

- Flexor tendon • Extensor tendon • Complex injuries • Skin grafts • Local flaps • Free tissue transfer
- Fascial flaps • Integra

KEY POINTS

- Complex hand injuries are those involving simultaneous compromise to multiple tissue types.
- Effective treatment is oriented to the restoration of viability, stability, sensibility, pliability, and mobility.
- Repair must often be performed in a staged fashion, with separate consideration given to the recovery of soft-tissue coverage and tendon integrity.

INTRODUCTION: NATURE OF THE PROBLEM

Complex flexor and extensor tendon injuries are those with significant associated bony or soft-tissue compromise that require consideration of reconstructive techniques beyond those limited to the tendons alone. Such injuries specifically involve loss of stable coverage over the extensor and/or flexor tendon mechanisms, which may or may not include damage to the paratenon. The most common mechanism accounting for these injuries is acute trauma; however, they may also be attributable to infection, malignancy, thermal injury, congenital deformation, and vascular malformation. Regardless of the underlying mechanism, effective surgical treatment may be complicated because of the requirement to reconstruct not only the mechanical underpinnings of meaningful hand function but also the investing soft-tissue envelope that serves to protect and preserve such structures.

THERAPEUTIC OPTIONS AND/OR SURGICAL TECHNIQUES

The goals of surgical repair of a complex hand injury include the simultaneous restoration of viability, stability, sensibility, pliability, and mobility.

The process of successfully achieving these goals begins with fastidious initial consideration and cataloging of the tissue types involved, including skin, subcutaneous tissue, nerve, vascular infrastructure, bone and articular structures, and, of course, tendons. A full delineation of the compromised tissues in these complex injuries depends on 3 key interventions that must be executed before undertaking definitive restoration of soft-tissue coverage and tendon integrity:

1. Restoration of reliable vascularity. It is a self-evident point that appropriate vascularity to the injured area must be established to enable adequate healing and reconstruction. When vascular compromise is noted at the time of injury, it must be addressed immediately, often on an emergent basis. A full discussion regarding approaches to revascularization and replantation is beyond the scope of this article, however, and is not further addressed here.
2. Stabilization of wound bed. All frankly devitalized tissues must be completely resected from the wound bed, both to provide an appropriate picture of what has been lost and to prevent downstream infection and excessive scar contracture once reconstruction has commenced.

[a] Division of Plastic Surgery, Harvard Medical School, Brigham and Women's Hospital, 75 Francis Street, Boston, MA 02114, USA; [b] Department of Orthopedic Surgery, Harvard Medical School, Brigham and Women's Hospital, 75 Francis Street, Boston, MA 02114, USA
* Corresponding author.
E-mail address: mcarty@partners.org

Hand Clin 29 (2013) 283–293
http://dx.doi.org/10.1016/j.hcl.2013.02.010
0749-0712/13/$ – see front matter © 2013 Elsevier Inc. All rights reserved.

The ability to establish a stable wound bed may require serial debridements during the first several days after injury, particularly in the case of severe crush and/or thermal injuries, which may demonstrate significant evolution of the apparent zone of injury over time. This process is often facilitated by the adjunctive use of negative pressure wound therapy.

3. Reestablishment of skeletal stability. When a significant skeletal or articular injury is a part of the overall injury pattern, it must be stabilized before coverage and/or tendon repair. Rigid stabilization typically permits earlier rehabilitation but may require more dissection and may change the options for soft-tissue coverage (ie, the fixation itself may require coverage beyond what the injured tissues alone required).

Once vascular, wound bed, and skeletal stabilities have been established, a definitive plan for complex reconstruction may be formulated effectively. In injuries in which the degree of soft-tissue loss overlying the area of concomitant tendon compromise precludes the possibility of linear closure, judgment is required to determine if primary tendon repair or grafting is likely to be superior to a staged reconstruction with interval placement of silicone rods until soft-tissue coverage is stable, followed by delayed tendon grafting. In general, staged reconstruction in these combined injuries is advisable, based on the conflicting requirements for success for soft-tissue reconstruction and tendon reconstruction, namely, the necessity for strict immobilization in the former and aggressive mobilization in the latter. In addition, simultaneous healing of the soft-tissue envelope and repaired/reconstructed tendon increases the likelihood of significant adhesions developing between these structures in the ensuing complex scar. If simultaneous soft-tissue and tendon reconstructions are undertaken, it should be expected that downstream tenolysis and capsulectomy may be required to achieve maximal functional benefit.

Restoration of Soft-Tissue Coverage

The principal objective of soft-tissue restoration is to provide stable coverage that is thin, pliable, sensate, and able to offer a gliding surface to permit appropriate excursion of the underlying tendon mechanisms. The critical determinant in guiding selection of the appropriate reconstructive modality is the condition of the paratenon, which normally serves as a well-vascularized investment to the tendon mechanism that simultaneously limits adhesion of surrounding tissues (**Table 1**).

Injuries in which the paratenon is intact and viable are generally amenable to simple skin grafting, as the integral lining typically serves as an excellent bed for graft incorporation; this is a particularly good option in the scenario of multiple digit injury, which is not an uncommon circumstance. Small defects are most readily addressed through full-thickness grafts from the ipsilateral forearm; contralateral dorsal hand; or inguinal crease (for non-glabrous skin), contralateral hypothenar area, or either foot instep (for glabrous skin); larger defects, however, typically require split-thickness skin grafts that are most often harvested from the lateral thigh. Compression of the grafted bed with either a tie-over bolster dressing or negative pressure dressing for 1 week is furthermore recommended to obviate shear and seroma/hematoma formation at the operative site and thereby limit the potential for graft failure.

If neighboring digits are uninjured and can therefore serve as reconstructive reservoirs, local digital flaps represent another option for coverage in the setting of intact paratenon. These include cross-finger flaps for volar digital defects, neurovascular island (Littler) flaps for volar or lateral digital defects (**Fig. 1**), and reverse cross-finger flaps for dorsal digital defects. The neurovascular island flap may be particularly useful for defects involving surfaces for which sensibility plays a more important functional role, such as the volar thumb pad and the lateral aspects of the border digits. Additional options for volar digital defects with intact palm integrity include thenar flaps (for radial digits) and hypothenar flaps (for ulnar digits), which provide excellent reconstructive substrates for pad loss but require a 2-staged operative plan. In summary, local digital flaps are versatile but, relative to simple skin grafts, must be carefully considered in terms of potential donor site morbidity and technical complexity.

Injuries in which the paratenon has been lost rarely successfully incorporate grafts directly and when they do are inherently plagued by problems of tendon adhesion. Under such circumstances, the re-creation of an adequate gliding surface is of paramount importance in promoting optimal functional recovery; reconstructive modalities that include a component that resists adhesion at the tendon surface interface are therefore indicated. Toward this end, reconstructive flaps that incorporate a fascial constituent (fascial flaps) represent an ideal option for the reconstruction of such complex defects. A host of local, regional, and distant fascial flaps have been described, providing a versatile armamentarium from which the reconstructive surgeon may draw to tackle these difficult injuries. Although a detailed review of all fascial flap options is beyond the scope of this article, the authors present here an overview of the various options that are available.

Selection of the appropriate fascial flap for reconstruction is determined by several factors including the availability of donor site, patient preference, and surgeon technical prowess; when all things are equal, however, the primary determinant of flap selection is the location of the defect on the injured hand. Specific flap options by anatomic location are described in the following.

Digital defects

Small defects involving the fingers may be addressed via venous flow-through flaps harvested from the volar wrist base. These flaps hinge on the "arterialization" of superficial veins in the flap substance that must be coapted to one or more digital arteries at the time of repair. Venous flow-through flaps typically involve little donor site morbidity and are technically straightforward; however, they require microsurgical prowess and may be characterized by significant venous congestion during the arterialization process.[1]

First web space and thumb defects

Small defects involving the first web space or thumb base are generally amenable to coverage via the locally available first dorsal metacarpal artery (FDMA) flap, which is easily dissected and has minimal associated donor site morbidity.[2] For larger defects or those that include compromise of the FDMA territory, the reversed pedicled radial forearm flap (RFF) represents an excellent alternative for thin and pliable coverage, particularly when harvested as a fascia-only substrate[3] (**Fig. 2**); however, adequacy of ulnar arterial inflow to the hand must be confirmed before obligatory sacrifice of the radial system for this flap. Both flaps offer the advantage of straightforward operative technique without the need for microsurgical anastomoses.

Dorsal hand and/or palm defects

Small to moderate-sized defects of the dorsal hand and palm are often amenable to coverage via regional pedicled fascial flap options including the reversed RFF, the reversed ulnar forearm flap,[4] and the posterior interosseous flap,[5] all of which may be performed without the aid of microsurgical intervention (**Fig. 3**). Defects that involve most of the dorsum or palm typically require more coverage than is available from these regional options and therefore necessitate the use of distant flaps that can provide more tissue. In the absence of microsurgical capability, the groin flap represents a tried and true pedicled option that is reliable and technically straightforward; however, it requires a staged

approach to repair, is limited primarily to dorsal hand defects, and generally must undergo subsequent debulking. Alternatively, a variety of fascial free flaps have been described for hand reconstruction and include the temporoparietal fascial (TPF) flap,[6] tensor fascia lata flap,[7] dorsalis pedis flap,[8] anterolateral thigh flap,[9] lateral arm flap,[10] serratus anterior flap,[11] and dorsal thoracic flap,[12] among others. All such flaps are significantly more technically demanding than pedicled options and require the appropriate facility infrastructure to support microsurgical intervention. Among the options available, the TPF offers perhaps the thinnest and most pliable free tissue substrate and has the added advantage of being transferred in an innervated fashion to permit restoration of sensibility[13] (**Fig. 4**); however, it is characterized by a challenging harvest with the potential for conspicuous alopecia and should be undertaken with caution.

Beyond autologous flap options, there is emerging evidence that there may be a role for the use of dermal regeneration templates such as Integra (Integra Life Sciences Corporation, Plainsboro, NJ, USA) in the treatment of complex hand injuries.[14,15] These bilayer wound matrices offer the potential to form a pseudofascial interface over denuded tendons that may be resistant to tendon adhesion and form a stable base for subsequent delayed split-thickness skin grafting. When successful, this approach has avoided the need for pedicled or free flap reconstruction, and has been used for both small and large hand defects. Data regarding long-term clinical outcomes are not yet available, however.

Regardless of the reconstructive modality used to restore soft-tissue integrity, meticulous postoperative care is essential to the success of the repair. The operative hand must remain elevated as much as is tolerated by the patient, ideally continuously for at least the first week after intervention. Strict immobilization via splinting is critical for appropriate healing for the first 7 to 10 days after repair, after which gentle passive and active range of motion exercises may be instituted under the watchful eye of a qualified hand therapist. Antibiotic prophylaxis is generally recommended for 1 week after reconstitution of the soft-tissue envelope, particularly in the case of open wounds that were previously heavily contaminated. For patients who have undergone repair via free tissue transfer, fastidious postoperative flap monitoring via clinical examination, Doppler monitoring and/or cutaneous tissue oximetry is warranted for 5 to 7 days; in such patients, the authors additionally advocate low-dose aspirin therapy for 4 weeks postoperatively, after which such therapy may be discontinued.

Table 1
Representative soft-tissue coverage options for complex hand injuries

Condition/Location	Operative Modality	Acronym/Eponym	Defect Size	Flap Type	Microsurgical	Advantages	Disadvantages
I. Paratenon intact							
A. Digits	Split-thickness/full-thickness skin graft	STSG/FTSG	Variable	N/A	No	Technical ease	Conspicuous donor site
	Cross-finger flap	None	Small	Pedicled local	No	Technical ease	Two-stage procedure, obligatory skin graft at harvest site
	Thenar/hypothenar flap	None	Small	Pedicled local	No	Technical ease	Two-stage procedure, obligatory skin graft at harvest site
	Neurovascular island flap	Littler flap	Small to moderate	Pedicled local	No	Sensate coverage	Donor site morbidity, obligatory skin graft at harvest site
B. Dorsum and Palm	Split-thickness/full-thickness skin graft	STSG/FTSG	Variable	N/A	No	Technical ease	Conspicuous donor site
II. Paratenon lost							
A. Digits	Venous flow-through flap	None	Small	Free	Yes	Minimal donor site morbidity	Venous congestion, variable success rate
	Dermal regeneration template with skin graft	None	Variable	N/A	No	Technical ease, versatility	Conspicuous donor site
B. First web space and thumb	First dorsal metacarpal artery flap	FDMA	Small	Pedicled local	No	Technical ease	Limited flap size
	Reversed radial forearm fascial flap	RFF	Moderate	Pedicled regional	No	Technical ease	Conspicuous donor site, sacrifice of radial inflow
	Dermal regeneration template with skin graft	None	Variable	N/A	No	Technical ease, versatility	Conspicuous donor site

			Size	Type	Sensate	Advantages	Disadvantages
C. Dorsal hand and palm	Reversed radial forearm fascial flap	RFF	Moderate	Pedicled regional	No	Technical ease	Conspicuous donor site, sacrifice of radial inflow
	Reversed ulnar forearm fascial flap	UFF	Moderate	Pedicled regional	No	Technical ease	Conspicuous donor site, sacrifice of ulnar inflow
	Posterior interosseous artery flap	PIA	Moderate	Pedicled regional	No	Preservation of radial system	Conspicuous donor site, technical difficulty
	Groin flap	None	Large	Pedicled distant	No	Technical ease	Bulky contour frequently requires revision, staged repair
	Temporoparietal fascial flap	TPF	Large	Free	Yes	Maximal thinness, potential for sensibility	Technical difficulty, donor site alopecia
	Tensor fascia lata flap	TFL	Large	Free	Yes	Technical ease	Conspicuous donor site, variable gait disturbance
	Dorsalis pedis flap	DP	Large	Free	Yes	Maximal thinness	Donor site irritation and conspicuousness
	Anterolateral thigh flap	ALT	Large	Free	Yes	Technical ease	Bulky contour frequently requires revision
	Lateral arm flap	LA	Large	Free	Yes	Technical ease	Bulky contour frequently requires revision
	Serratus anterior flap	SA	Large	Free	Yes	Inconspicuous donor site	Technical difficulty, potential for scapular winging
	Dorsal thoracic flap	DT	Large	Free	Yes	Minimal donor site morbidity	Obligatory position change during procedure
	Dermal regeneration template with skin graft	None	Variable	N/A	No	Technical ease, versatility	Conspicuous donor site
D. Special case	Vascularized composite allotransplantation	VCA	Variable	Free	Yes	No donor site	Obligatory lifelong immunosuppression

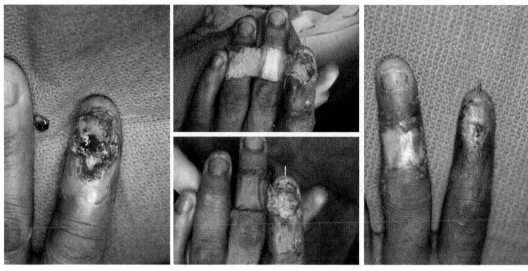

Fig. 1. Cross-finger flap reconstruction of the digit. A 46-year-old man sustained severe crush injury to the left index fingertip, resulting in avulsion of dorsal soft-tissue coverage overlying the distal interphalangeal joint and extensor tendon disruption. Repair was performed using a cross-finger flap from the unaffected ipsilateral long finger. Four-week follow-up photos demonstrate ongoing healing at the injury site and mild hypopigmentation at the donor site. (*Courtesy of* C. Sampson, MD.)

Restoration of Tendon Integrity

The treatment options for tendon injury include primary repair, secondary repair, immediate reconstruction with tendon graft, staged tendon reconstruction, and tendon transfer. When direct repair of adequate tendon is possible, that is typically performed; as referenced previously, however, more complex tendon injuries that occur in the presence of concomitant compromise of the overlying soft tissues generally require staged reconstruction; this is particularly true for injuries that involve the flexor mechanism, since the flexor tenolysis that would be expected after a single-staged repair is more complex and challenging than the extensor mechanism given the presence of the flexor pulley system and the higher likelihood of tendon rupture after tenolysis.[16] In such injuries, therefore, it is advisable to perform initial reconstruction of the flexor sheath pulleys system and placement of a silicone rod at the time of soft-tissue coverage, followed by definitive tendon reconstruction via interposition grafting or tendon transfer 3 to 6 months afterward.

For injuries involving the extensor mechanism, there are instances that an interposition tendon graft or tendon transfer may be performed in conjunction with soft-tissue coverage in a single-staged fashion. In such cases, it must once again be emphasized that downstream tenolysis and/or other secondary procedures are most likely warranted (**Fig. 5**). In instances in which a staged approach is selected, the operative technique is

similar to that of similar injuries involving the flexor surface, with the additional caveat that care must be taken to restore the integrity of the extensor retinaculum.[17]

Regardless of timing, when a free tendon graft is chosen, the most common donor candidates include the palmaris longus and plantaris. Toe extensors are also selected in settings where multiple tendons may be needed for the roughly 10% of patients with an absent palmaris longus tendon. Redundant tendons on the dorsum of the hand such as the extensor indicis proprius and extensor digit minimi also can serve as tendon graft donors. Lastly, in a percentage of these injuries, there may be adequate tendon material in tissue that would otherwise be discarded, as in the case of a nonreconstructable digit.

Several available options for soft-tissue coverage have the option of incorporating vascularized tendon components. These singled-staged reconstructions have the advantage of using normal, vascular tendon components that are less likely to adhere to the transferred tissue. However, the number of tendon elements available is limited in size, shape, and orientation and may not be applicable to many defects.

Special Case: Vascularized Composite Allotransplantation

During the past 20 years, the notion of vascularized composite allotransplantation (VCA) for the treatment of severe upper extremity injuries has moved

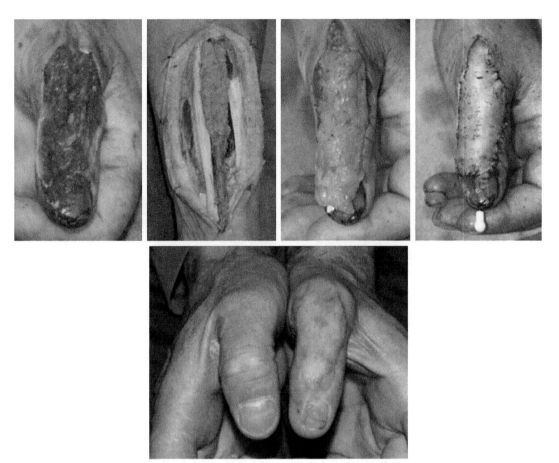

Fig. 2. Pedicled radial forearm fascial flap reconstruction to the thumb. A 57-year-old man carpenter sustained an industrial router injury to the left thumb, including loss of dorsal skin and most of the extensor pollicis longus, with exposure of the underlying proximal phalanx. Repair was performed via a reversed radial forearm fascial flap over an interposition tendon graft reconstruction. A split-thickness skin graft was applied to restore skin integrity. His appearance at 8 months is depicted. (*From* Carty MJ, Taghinia A, Upton J. Fascial flap reconstruction of the hand: a single surgeon's 30-year experience. Plast Reconstr Surg 2010;125:953; with permission.)

from the realm of science fiction to scientific fact; to date, more than 70 hand transplants have been performed worldwide. In general, the functional outcomes witnessed among hand transplant recipients have been better than expected, and the morbidity of lifelong immunosuppression has been less than anticipated. The degree to which VCA may be used to reconstruct partial hand defects has yet to be fully explored. At present, few centers performing VCA procedures would consent to perform an allotransplantation procedure for an isolated partial hand injury; however, patients who require concomitant VCA for other corporeal defects may be candidates for simultaneous hand reconstruction. In the authors' institution, they performed one such case to date that involved a patient with severe facial and extremity thermal injuries. The patient underwent full facial allotransplantation and simultaneous repair of a complex right dorsal hand injury via a composite RFF harvested from the donor. This repair included resurfacing of the entirety of the recipient's dorsal hand, as well as simultaneous reconstruction of several extensor tendons through a combination of a palmaris (which was included in the donor RFF) and multiple extensor tendon interposition allografts (**Fig. 6**). The patient has subsequently achieved remarkable improvement in hand function without evidence of rejection. The indications for interventions of this type for complex hand injuries, although presently uncertain, will undoubtedly continue to be defined and revised in the coming years.

CLINICAL OUTCOMES

Because of the diverse nature of these complex injuries, it is difficult to make general statements

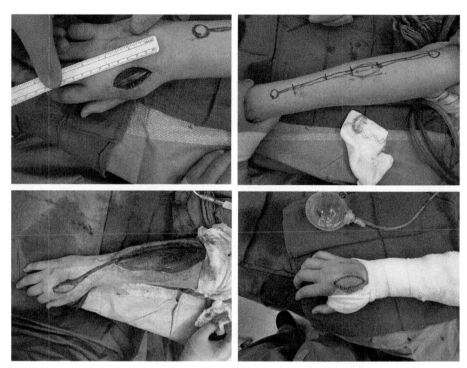

Fig. 3. Posterior interosseous artery flap reconstruction of a dorsal hand defect. A 28-year-old woman suffered a dorsal hand crush injury resulting in a large dorsal hand hematoma and necrosis of the overlying skin and extensor paratenon. The necrotic tissues were debrided, and a pedicled posterior interosseous artery flap was elevated and transposed into the ensuing defect.

concerning the clinical outcomes of reconstruction. As one would intuit, the more severe the injury and the greater the number of constituent tissues involved, the greater the challenge to restore normal hand function. The highest likelihood for meaningful recovery arises from a confluence of factors including appropriate acute management, a principles-based approach to reconstruction, and devout patient compliance with recommended hand therapy. The spectrum of potential clinical outcomes is at least partially illustrated in the case examples included in this review.

COMPLICATIONS AND CONCERNS

The treatment of complex hand injuries is challenging and, as expected, is characterized by a host of potential complications above and beyond those of more mundane hand procedures. Among the possible complications, the following warrant specific mention.

Repair Failure

Failure of primary tendon repairs is unfortunately still expected with current repair techniques, which is more often an issue with digital flexor tendons than extensors or wrist level tendons. Estimations of the risk of failure due to overt rupture

or significant gap formation vary; rates approaching 20% have been reported even with current techniques.[18] Although no comparative studies have been published to date on the subject, rupture rates may be lower with combined injuries given the propensity for increased scarring that exists.

Technical Difficulty

These injuries are challenging and are ideally addressed by using a wide variety of techniques, not all of which are in the armamentarium of every hand surgeon. The vast majority of these injuries have multiple options for reconstruction without a clear gold standard; there are few controlled trials addressing superiority of one technique over another. When faced with equally appropriate options, therefore, operative surgeons should generally select the one with which they are most familiar and facile. There may be occasions in which consultation with a colleague with a different skill set may be helpful.

Donor Site Morbidity

The choice of reconstruction must include consideration for the morbidity at the donor site, which varies significantly among the various

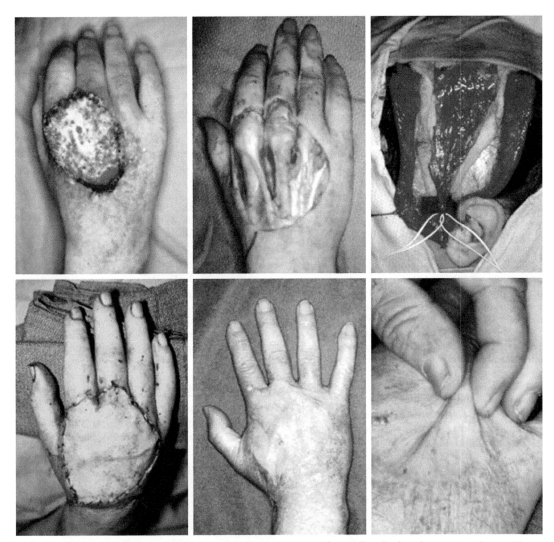

Fig. 4. Chronicle of the first reported case using temporoparietal fascial flap for hand reconstruction. A 56-year-old man presented with large dorsal hand squamous cell carcinoma. Resection resulted in a large dorsal wound with exposed bone and extensor loss. A temporoparietal fascial flap was harvested and inset with an overlying split-thickness skin graft. At 30-year follow-up, the patient demonstrates excellent flap contour and suppleness. (*From* Carty MJ, Taghinia A, Upton J. Fascial flap reconstruction of the hand: a single surgeon's 30-year experience. Plast Reconstr Surg 2010;125:953; with permission.)

options discussed (see **Table 1**). A frank discussion of the potential complications associated with each considered reconstructive method may lead to a superior selection for a given individual (ie, a patient may have a strong preference to limit donor sites to the ipsilateral arm after a major injury).

Need for Secondary Procedures

Secondary procedures are not only commonly required but they are also intrinsic to many of the techniques described earlier. Discussing this

with the patient early on, including a detailed overview of timing, is critical. As mentioned previously, the need for tenolysis is expected with many of these injuries. Prerequisites for tenolysis include a supple digit, failure to advance further in motion, and a patient who demonstrates the ability to actively participate. Tenolysis surgery should be performed through supple, not inflamed, skin. Scars with erythema and firmness to touch are still maturing, and the authors recommend against proceeding in this setting. Timing is a major consideration; there is no clear evidence-based answer, but it is infrequent that these conditions

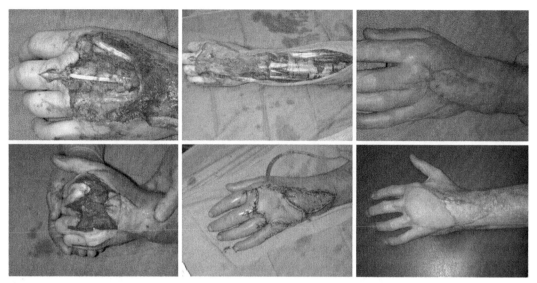

Fig. 5. Regional flap reconstruction of dorsal hand defect with simultaneous single-stage extensor tendon repair via interposition graft. A 45-year-old man suffered a degloving injury to the dorsum of his left hand, resulting in a large soft-tissue defect and disruption of the long finger extensor mechanism. Initial repair with a concomitant interposition tendon graft, adipofascial flap, and skin graft was complicated by significant contracture requiring downstream scar release, capsulectomy, and an additional pedicled ulnar forearm flap. Six-month follow-up demonstrates stable coverage and improved range of motion.

are met before 3 to 4 months after the initial injury/surgery. Given the high rate of previously unidentified flexor tendon ruptures that occur with tenolysis, patients also need to approach this as a major surgical undertaking.

Flap Debulking

In general, the reconstructive principal is to replace "like with like"; however, this is not always possible. In the hand, this frequently leads to the

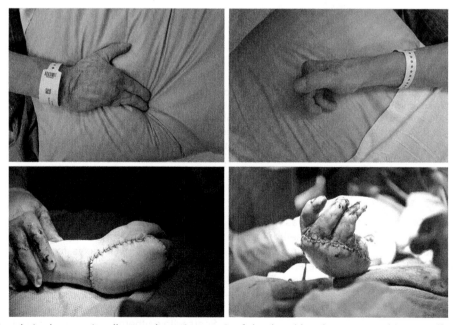

Fig. 6. Vascularized composite allotransplantation repair of the dorsal hand. A 32-year-old man suffered severe thermal injuries to the face and bilateral hands, resulting in loss of the extensors to this right index and long finger and unstable dorsal hand coverage. He underwent full face allotransplantation and simultaneous transplantation of a large radial forearm flap from the donor to the dorsal right hand, in conjunction with interposition repair of the deficient extensor tendons. (*Courtesy of* B. Pomahac, MD.)

need for debulking procedures. Indications for debulking can include both aesthetic concerns and functional limitations. Traditionally, debulking has been performed through serial excision procedures over the course of several months. Newer techniques, however, now open up the possibility for single-staged debulking via liposuction or direct tissue excision followed by reapplication of the flap skin as a skin graft.

SUMMARY

Complex injuries of the hand represent a challenging clinical entity. Although these injuries are diverse and are therefore not amenable to a strict treatment algorithm, a thoughtful approach to care can be formulated through the application of basic reconstructive principles. These include initial wound and skeletal stabilization, followed by concomitant or staged restoration of soft-tissue coverage and tendon integrity. With appropriate treatment, patients suffering from these wounds can be expected to achieve a level of functional recovery commensurate with the severity of their initial injury.

REFERENCES

1. Rozen WM, Leong J. Arterialized venous flow-through flaps with dual discontiguous venous drainage: a new modification to improve flap survival. Plast Reconstr Surg 2012;130:229e–31e.
2. Foucher G, Braun JB. A new island flap transfer from the dorsum of the index to the thumb. Plast Reconstr Surg 1979;63:344–9.
3. Taghinia AH, Carty M, Upton J. Fascial flaps for hand reconstruction. J Hand Surg Am 2010;35:1351–5.
4. Becker C, Gilbert A. The ulnar flap. Handchir Mikrochir Plast Chir 1988;20:180–3 [in German].
5. Zancolli EA, Angrigiani C. Posterior interosseous island forearm flap. J Hand Surg Br 1988;13:130–5.
6. Upton J, Rogers C, Durham-Smith G, et al. Clinical applications of the free temporoparietal flaps in hand reconstruction. J Hand Surg Am 1986;11:475–83.
7. Nahai F, Silverton JS, Hill H, et al. The tensor fascia lata musculocutaneous flap. Ann Plast Surg 1978;1:372–9.
8. Ritz M, Mahendru S, Somia N, et al. The dorsalis pedis fascial flap. J Reconstr Microsurg 2009;25:313–7.
9. Adani R, Tarallo L, Marcoccio I, et al. Hand reconstruction using the thin anterolateral thigh flap. Plast Reconstr Surg 2005;116:467–73.
10. Song R, Song Y, Yu Y, et al. The upper arm free flap. Clin Plast Surg 1982;9:27–35.
11. Flugel A, Heitmann C, Kehrer A, et al. Defect coverage of the hand with the free serratus fascial flap. Handchir Mikrochir Plast Chir 2005;37:186–92 [in German].
12. Colen LB, Pessa JE, Potparic Z, et al. Reconstruction of the extremity with the dorsal thoracic fascia free flap. Plast Reconstr Surg 1998;101:738–44.
13. Carty MJ, Taghinia A, Upton J. Fascial flap reconstruction of the hand: a single surgeon's 30 year experience. Plast Reconstr Surg 2010;125:953–62.
14. Weigert R, Chougri H, Casoli V. Management of severe hand injuries with Integra dermal regeneration template. J Hand Surg Eur 2011;36:185–93.
15. Rizzo M. The use of Integra in hand and upper extremity surgery. J Hand Surg Am 2010;37:583–6.
16. Eggli S, Dietsche A, Eggli S, et al. Tenolysis after combined digital injuries in zone II. Ann Plast Surg 2005;55:266–71.
17. Kawakatsu M, Ishikawa K, Terai T. Importance of the reconstruction of the extensor retinaculum after injury. J Plast Surg Hand Surg 2011;45:252–4.
18. Su BW, Solomons M, Barrow A, et al. Device for zone-II flexor tendon repair. A multicenter, randomized, blinded, clinical trial. J Bone Joint Surg Am 2005;87:923–35.

Current Flexor and Extensor Tendon Motion Regimens: A Summary

Sean P. Clancy, OTR/L, CHT[a,b,c],*, Daniel P. Mass, MD[d,e]

KEYWORDS

- Controlled stress • Flexor tendon rehabilitation • Extensor tendon rehabilitation
- Early passive motion • Early active motion

KEY POINTS

- After flexor tendon repair, early passive digital flexion regime is used popularly. Early active digital flexion is advocated increasingly in recent years following a strong tendon repair and possibly results in better recovery.
- Following extensor tendon repair, some therapists and surgeons use early tendon mobilization, but others use passive motion or immobilization. Whether the extensor tendon should be moved actively or passively, or immobilized, is controversial.
- Application of the "right" force to move the digits is important to moving the repaired tendon while avoiding repair rupture. "Proper" positioning of the joints is important to reducing tension in the tendon.
- An ideal protocol improves gliding of a repaired tendon, avoids repair rupture or gapping potential, and leads to a better functional return.
- A variety of protocols are available, which should be selected and modified according to the extent of trauma to the tendon, strength of the tendon repair, and compliance of the patient.

The idea of applying controlled stress to a repaired tendon has existed for nearly 40 years.[1,2] Recently, improved modern repair techniques, with understanding of the physiologic concepts and technologic advancements, repair strengths have improved our ability to move tendons early.[3–18] Surgeons and therapists are currently assessing the available evidence in search of the perfect recipe for appropriate stress. This article summarizes the current flexor and extensor motion regimens.

Regimens or protocols are often misused as an absolute guide to rehabilitation. This is an inappropriate way to rehabilitate an individual with a tendon injury. The regimens are to be used as a guide to practice. The exact methods should be decided based on communication and teamwork between the patient, surgeon, and therapist. Deviation from a regimen is a common practice because each individual patient presents with specific factors that can affect the decision of use of specific components of regimens. It is possible to use multiple aspects of different protocols to fit the patient's needs or physiologic profile change.

FLEXOR TENDON REGIMENS

Repaired flexor tendons present specific challenges to the patient and therapist. **Fig. 1**

[a] Hand Therapy Program, University of Chicago Medicine, 5841 South Maryland, Chicago, IL 60637-1470, USA; [b] Physical Therapy Residency Program, University of Chicago Medicine, 5841 South Maryland, Chicago, IL 60637-1470, USA; [c] Hand Therapy Clinic, MC 1081 DCAM 4a, 5841 South Maryland, Chicago, IL, USA; [d] Department of Orthopaedic Surgery and Rehabilitation Medicine, Orthopaedic Surgery, University of Chicago Pritzker School of Medicine, University of Chicago Medicine, 5841 South Maryland, MC 3079, Chicago, IL 60637, USA; [e] Hand and Microsurgery Fellowship Program, University of Chicago Medicine, 5841 South Maryland, MC 3079, Chicago, IL 60637, USA
* Corresponding author. Hand Therapy Clinic, MC 1081 DCAM 4a, 5841 South Maryland, Chicago, IL.
E-mail address: Sean.Clancy@uchospitals.edu

Hand Clin 29 (2013) 295–309
http://dx.doi.org/10.1016/j.hcl.2013.03.002

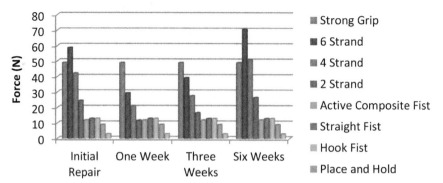

Fig. 1. Comparison of estimated stress of therapy interventions used in some flexor tendon exercise regimens and the strengths of 2-, 4-, and 6-strand core suture repairs. It does not take into consideration improvements in suture material or the multiple factors experienced in a patient. It is obvious that use of a power grasp may result in rupture or gapping throughout the scale. This graph includes information from Dr Strickland. (*Data from* Refs.[6,10,19,44])

illustrates different rehabilitative controlled stress management tools available to the therapist and the strengths of 2-, 4- and 6-strand repairs. This information is important to all experience levels of therapists to truly understand the application of controlled stress on a patient's repair site. Most surgeons now prefer to initiate motion exercises 4 to 6 days after surgery to avoid the period of marked edema and pain. The rehabilitation persists for 8–12 weeks or even longer.

There are 3 general types of flexor tendon protocols: immobilization, early passive motion (EPM), and early active motion (EAM). Immobilization protocols are commonly found and are generally accepted. Immobilization protocols are used with children from birth to 10 years old and patients who cannot cognitively comprehend other regimens. Early passive and active regimens are the focus of this section. Studies have shown that early mobilization of tendons can improve the healing process and the strength of the repair.[1,2,8,10,17–19] EPM protocols were developed more than 35 years ago based on a 2-strand repair. The protocols were designed based on Duran and Houser's theory that 3 to 5 mm of tendon excursion can decrease tendon adhesion formation.[1] These protocols remain a relevant option for the individual interested in rehabilitating patients. In a 2005 journal article, Groth studied practice patterns for flexor tendon rehabilitation. She found that the Kleinert and Duran protocols have remained in use throughout the midwest United States with roughly two-thirds of the participants reporting its use.[20] Although many aspects of flexor tendon repair have been improved through research, there remain situations in which a 2-strand repair is necessary. Both protocols begin with basic wound care, edema control, and a custom-fabricated dorsal blocking orthosis (DBO).

The original Kleinert and Duran protocols were modified over the years by hand therapists. The Kleinert protocol is less used nowadays. The Kleinert protocol originally had a splint made of cast material and rubber band traction passively flexing the proximal interphalangeal (PIP) joints only.[2] The wrist was positioned in 45° of flexion and 10° to 20° of metacarpophalangeal (MP) and PIP flexion. The Kleinert protocol has changed with the wrist positioned at 20° to 30° of flexion and the MP joints 50° to 70°. The greatest change from the original orthosis was to place a palmar bar to include the distal interphalangeal (DIP) joints into composite flexion. This can be accomplished by a prefabricated flexor tendon brace or fabrication of the components by a therapist.[21] The initial exercises are passive composite and noncomposite passive finger motion within the orthosis. The patient also completes active extension against rubber band traction 50 times a waking hour. Place and holds are initiated at 3 weeks. At 4 weeks, the DBO is refabricated with the wrist in neutral. Differential gliding, isolated flexor digitorum superficialis (FDS) exercises, and passive interphalangeal extension stretches are added. The wrist is exercised at midrange. During the sixth week, the DBO is discontinued. Composite wrist and digital motion, gentle passive extension exercises, and proximal blocking exercises are initiated. The small finger may not tolerate proximal blocking and the therapist risks potential tendon rupture. This technique is not recommended for the small finger. In the seventh week light resistive exercises (PREs) starts, with progression to work simulation in the eighth week. Application of the Kleinert protocol requires good custom orthotic fabrication skills and experience with recognizing tendon adhesions. The use of a rubber band leads to digital joint flexion contracture. Kleinert protocol is an early method and complex. Now fewer and fewer surgeons use this protocol.

The Duran protocol originally used a dorsal blocking orthosis with rubber band traction.[1] The modified versions of the Duran protocol eliminated the rubber band traction opting to use a strap to hold the digits in extension when not exercising. The current protocol for the custom DBO is 20° of wrist flexion, the MP joints at 70°, and the interphalangeal joints in neutral.[21] This modified Duran protocol is still used in many units in the United States. Once edema is managed, the patient can complete repetitions of noncomposite PIP and DIP passive flexion/extension. These exercises are followed by composite passive motion in both planes. All exercises are completed inside the DBO and are completed every 2 waking hours. This treatment regimen continues until 3.5 weeks when the patient is allowed to complete an active composite flexion/extension fist in the DBO. Composite wrist and digital flexion/extension exercises are completed at 4.5 weeks outside the DBO. Hook fist exercises customized with movement from the hook position to full interphalangeal extension is completed. Wrist flexion extension with a composite fist is also initiated at this time. The DBO is discontinued at 5.5 weeks. Passive extension stretching and proximal blocking exercises are added to the treatment regimen at 6 weeks. The small finger should not participate in the blocking program for reasons previously stated in the Kleinert protocol. The 8-week point marks the addition of PREs (see **Fig. 1**; **Fig. 2**, **Table 1**).

EARLY ACTIVE MOTION REGIMENS

Early active motion (EAM) protocols differ from EPM protocols in many ways. The most significant

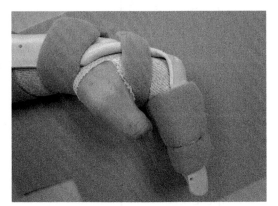

Fig. 2. The Duran protocol orthosis in its modified form.

difference is that the excursion imparted on the tendon is completed with an active contraction of a muscle unit. The EAM was first introduced by a group of surgeons in Belfast. Now many units use EAM regimes. Korstanje and colleagues[24] measured tendon excursion of healthy subjects using ultrasonography. They found that the absolute and relative excursion of the tendons was greater with active motion protocols. There are many early active protocols in the literature.[22,25–38] These protocols attempt to control the active motion by different means. All the protocols featured in this section use a DBO with configurations in varying joint positions (see **Table 4**). EAM is an ill-defined categorization. It is debatable what exact criterion is necessary to describe the term "active". The premise of this article is to present a summary of early motion regimens useful for tendon rehabilitation. Any mobilization other than complete passive excursion of the tendon is considered active.

An international group of regimens is described below in this section. The Indiana,[26,39] Mass,[36] and Nantong[34] protocols are briefly discussed and described. These protocols require at least a 4-strand repair or greater, a compliant motivated patient, and moderate to minimal edema. A flexor tendon injury that is complicated by concomitant injuries requiring immobilization precludes EAM application. The Indiana tenodesis protocol differs from the Mass and Nantong protocols by using place and hold exercise to stress the repair site. The tools used by the hand therapist vary initially. The Indiana tenodesis program elicits tendon motion through the modified Duran exercise followed by a specifically described place and hold exercise. The Mass protocol uses the modified Duran exercises followed by active contraction of the patient's musculotendinous unit. The Nantong protocol uses full active extension and passive flexion followed by active composite fisting through half or two-thirds of the full flexion range (eg, partial or limited range active digital flexion) in the first a few weeks. For cases involving FDS and FDP repairs, differential gliding may be used. The initiation of movement in the initial stages of an EAM regimen is threefold: (1) tendon repairs through active excursion are stressed safely; (2) adhesion formation is abated; (3) elasticity of other soft tissues is maintained. All protocols involving flexor tendon repairs require astute management of edema and wound site integrity.

Progression of the controlled stress also differs between protocols. The Indiana tenodesis protocol does not impart an active composite fist until 4 weeks. The Indiana methodology is to reduce stress on the repair to the fullest and impart the

Table 1
Early passive motion regimens

Early Passive Regimen	Initial/Protected Phase	Protected Mobilization Phase	Progressive Resistance Phase	
	0–3 d	3–4 wk	4–6 wk	6–8 wk
Kleinert (modified)[2,21–23]	DBO fabricated Active extension exercises against rubber band traction in DBO. Rubber bands return digits to flexion (50 repetitions per waking hour)	3 wk: active composite fisting within DBO	4 wk: discontinue rubber band traction DBO (wrist neutral) Tendon gliding exercises, protected isolated FDS active gliding, and protected PIP/DIP passive extension stretches are initiated 5 wk: nonresistive blocking techniques	6 wk: discontinue DBO Resistive blocking exercises and light functional activities initiated 7 wk: unrestricted active and passive motion and light strengthening 8 wk: PREs
Duran (modified)[22,23]	DBO fabricated Duran exercise program: Noncomposite passive MP, PIP, and DIP range of motion followed by composite flexion of all digital joints (25 repetitions every 2 h)	3.5 wk: active composite fist in DBO	4.5: wk unprotected active composite wrist and digital flexion and extension outside DBO (25 repetitions every 2 waking hours) 5.5 wk: discontinue DBO	6 wk: proximal blocking (except fifth digit) Passive extension stretching initiated 8 wk: light strengthening

most effective excursion on the tendon to reduce adhesions. In a cadaveric study, Tanaka and colleagues[18] found that, when the wrist is in extension with the digits fully flexed, there was no tension. The tenodesis with place and hold is the main difference between this and the other EAM regimens presented in the article. The original protocol calls for 2 orthoses: an exercise orthosis and a DBO. The exercise orthosis uses a wrist hinge over the anatomic axis and allows for 30° of wrist extension. It is possible to create the DBO orthosis with a hinge and a removable block to use 1 dual-purpose orthosis and reduce possible patient confusion. A prospective study by Trumble and colleagues[40] found that EAM provided greater digital motion compared with EPM protocols in zone 2. The EAM protocol used was much like the Indiana tenodesis exercises. At 4 weeks the Indiana tenodesis is discontinued and the protocol continues a path similar to the other EAM protocols reported in this article.

The Mass protocol[36] also uses information gathered from sources similar to other EAM protocols but with a different approach. The DBO in this protocol places the wrist in 20° of wrist extension. Sandow and McMahon[41,42] published a study using a similar orthosis and protocol postoperatively. The wrist extension decreases the work of flexion of the tendon[12] and reduces tension on the repair site.[18] Active composite fisting is attempted through the available range after edema control measures and passive noncomposite and composite digital flexion. The repair remains protected by the DBO for 6 weeks. The MP joints are allowed to move to full extension with refabrication. This protocol was first published in 2005 by Coats and colleagues.[36] Although there are no studies publishing results on this exact protocol, it has been used successfully clinically. The Sandow and McMahon[41] study reported 71% good to excellent results in 73 tendons using the Strickland and Glogovac grading system.[19]

The Nantong Protocol[34] uses a 3-stage process to systematically achieve the prescribed goals. In the first 2.5 weeks, the goal is to achieve full extension of the PIP joints primarily and half to two-thirds of an active composite fist secondarily. This is conducted in an orthosis that is more protective and conservative than the previous protocols (see **Table 3**). In the second 2.5 weeks, the focus of the therapy is to achieve a full active composite fist. The DBO is refabricated to place the wrist in 30° of extension. During the next 2.5 weeks, the patient remains protected with the DBO until the sixth or seventh week. Light PREs and activities of daily life (ADL) are initiated. At 8 weeks, normal use of the hand may commence. The Nantong protocol uses a combination of ideas used to design the other EAM protocols and takes into consideration some of the complications of tendon repair in its implementation (**Figs. 3–7**, **Tables 2** and **3**).

In past two years, therapists and surgeons in Manchester, England, started to use a short DBO to protect only joints of the hand (with the DIP and PIP joints straight, and MP joint in mild flexion), leaving the wrist free to flex and moderately extend, The dorsal splint is fabricated so that further extension of the wrist beyond 45° is blocked by contact with the forearm. The proximal edge of the splint is flared gently and padded to prevent rubbing. They performed EAM after flexor tendon repair with multi-strand repair methods. No increases in repair rupture have been noted with the short DBO protection.

EXTENSOR TENDON REGIMENS

Commonalities between the repairs of extensor tendon and flexor tendon repairs are extrinsic

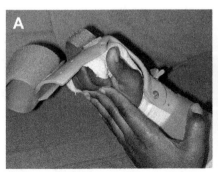
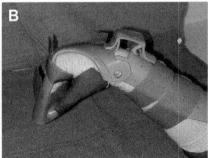

Fig. 3. (*A*) The Indiana tenodesis orthosis. A rigid thermoplastic block is used, which is removed for exercise and donned to revert from exercise orthosis to DBO. (*B*) The patient passively moves digits into composite flexion with the wrist blocked in 30° of extension. The patient then holds for 5 seconds. They then relax the wrist bringing the wrist into flexion.

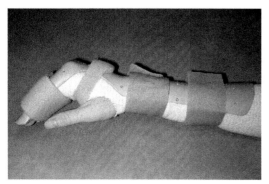

Fig. 4. The Mass regimen places the wrist in 20° of extension from the first postoperative visit.

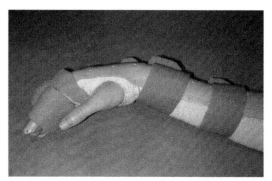

Fig. 6. The original Nantong regimen orthosis includes the thumb. The thumb portion can be left off with the compliant patient to protect from inadvertent pinching. The goal of the initial phase is full extension.

and intrinsic healing, repair strength increasing in response to controlled stress, and the presence of similar anatomic challenges. Extensor tendons differ anatomically and biomechanically from flexor tendons in their total cross-section areas, tendon excursion, intertendinous connections, and capacity of work.

Extensor tendon repairs pose their own difficulties with regard to rehabilitation. Immobilization was once the standard treatment. Immobilization continues to be used in many zones despite evidence that optimal outcomes are achieved with early motion protocols.[43] Immobilization remains the best care for injuries in zones I and II. Patients who are young or lack the cognition to comply with early motion protocols can receive immobilization protocols. The therapist must be aware of the characteristics of the stages of healing to properly manage the repaired extensor tendon. The symbiotic relationship between the referring surgeon and the hand therapy clinic assists in favorable outcomes. Early motion must be started preferably from 24 to 48 hours and no later than a week after surgery. The goals of the therapist are to apply the correct controlled stress to a repair site, avoid adhesion formation, and provent potential gapping at the repair site.

There are many extensor tendon early motion protocols and variations.[43] The short arc motion

protocol (SAM),[44,45] the immediate controlled active range of motion (ICAM),[46] an augmented zone V-VII protocol,[47] and the double reverse Kleinert protocol[48] are presented here. Some are practical, and a few are difficult to apply correctly. The protocols provide options for the hand clinic treating zone III to zone VII injuries. Often extensor tendons are perceived as easier rehabilitation targets than the flexor tendons. This premise is an unfortunate misconception. Patients undergoing extensor tendon rehabilitation are often the most difficult and intricate cases. This summary should be used in conjunction with independent study to completely understand the concepts to apply to the postoperative patient.

SAM was developed by Rosalyn Evans and first published in 1988 in the *Journal of Hand Therapy*.[43] The SAM protocol's genesis was based on Evans's experience battling the complications of injuries in zones III and IV. This protocol begins early postoperatively. It consists of 3 custom-fabricated orthoses. The first orthosis is static and immobilizes the PIP and DIP joints in 0° extension. The other 2 orthoses are for exercise. The patient removes the static orthosis and dons the

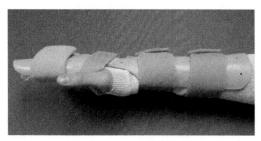

Fig. 5. The orthosis is remolded to allow 0° of MP extension in the sixth week in the Mass regimen.

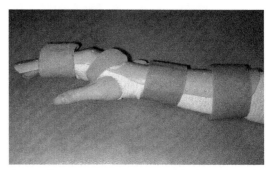

Fig. 7. The Nantong DBO is modified to place the wrist in 20° of extension during phase 2.

Table 2
Comparison of EAM regimens

Early AROM Protocols	Initial to 2.5 wk	3–4 wk	5–7 wk	8–12 wk
Indiana Tenodesis[26,39]	Fabricate custom DBO Modified Duran exercises Active place and holds in tenodesis orthosis	4 wk: tenodesis orthosis discontinued Unprotected active composite, straight, and hook fisting with wrist not exceeding neutral Active motion of the wrist with no digital involvement	5 wk: active composite wrist and digital flexion/extension 6 wk: DBO discontinued If necessary proximal blocking except small finger	8 wk: initiate PREs (the Indiana tenodesis protocol progresses treatment options as the tendon repair strengthens. The new exercises are completed as a compliment to the initial exercise in the order they are allowed)
Mass protocol at the University of Chicago Medicine[36]	Fabricate custom DBO Modified Duran exercises Passive composite fists Active composite fist gently through available range (in clinic)	Continue treatment encouraging increased AROM Take measures to decrease PIP joint extensor lag	6 wk: modify DBO MP joints to 0° extension Continue treatment encouraging increased AROM	8 wk: initiate PREs (During treatment, the patient may complete active composite fists during their home exercise program if determined appropriate by the surgeon)
Nantong protocol[34]	Fabricate custom DBO Full active extension and passive flexion Partial active composite flexion to 50%	2.5–3 wk: refabrication of DBO Protected active flexion/extension of digits through full range	6 wk: light return to ADL 6–7 wk: DBO discontinued	8 wk: initiate PREs (the modified Duran exercises can be used throughout the protocol if necessary. Passive motion precedes active exercise in all phases)

Abbreviation: AROM, active range of motion.

exercise orthoses every waking hour for 20 repetitions each. These exercises are completed in support of the principle of minimal active tension.[49] The SAM protocol strives to impart controlled stress to a specific area, in this case the central slip, to decrease the incidence of adhesions. It is pivotal that exhaustive patient education regarding this protocol be conducted to ensure compliance and success.

During the first 2 weeks of the initial exercise program, the wrist is held in 30° of extension. The MPs are supported by the patient's opposite hand, in slight or 0° flexion. The PIP blocking orthosis is supported by the patient's opposite hand ensuring the PIP joint is at 0° during the exercise. The patient is educated to complete the full available arc of motion and to hold the fully extended position briefly. The cadence of the exercise is slow and methodical. After 2 weeks, the PIP joint palmar blocking orthosis is remolded to allow for 40° of flexion. This is delayed if there is an extensor lag present. In the third week, the patient's PIP joint flexion block can be moved to 50° and advanced to 70° to 80° at the fourth week. If a lag is present, the therapist may half the incremental progression of the PIP joint orthosis angle. Patient reeducation on protocol compliance should be conducted regularly especially in lieu of the presence of an extensor lag. The fifth week begins a new phase in which the patient is allowed composite exercises and PREs. Discharge is possible to a home exercise program at 6 weeks. This protocol requires independent study before attempting it on a patient (**Fig. 8**A–E).

Table 3
Comparison of EPM and EAM custom orthoses

Regimen	Wrist Position	MP Joint	Interphalangeal Joint	Special Considerations
Early Passive Motion (EPM)				
Modified Kleinert[2,21–23]	20°–30° of flexion	50°–70° of flexion	0° of flexion	Either a PFT is fitted or fingernail hooks, palmar line guides, and rubber band traction are fabricated/applied
Modified Duran[22,23]	20° of flexion	65°–70° of flexion	0° of flexion	
Early Active Regimens (EAM)				
Indiana tenodesis[26,39]	20° of flexion	65°–70° of flexion	0° of flexion	Authors use 1 dual-purpose DBO protocol, which calls for a DBO and an exercise orthosis
Mass protocol at the University of Chicago Medicine[36]	20° of extension	70° of flexion	0° of flexion	MP joints are changed to 0° at 6 wk
Nantong protocol[34]	20°–30° of flexion	Slight to mild flexion 20°–30°	0° of flexion or slight flexion	Wrist position is changed to 20° of extension at 2.5 to 3 wk

The ICAM regimen[43,46,50] can be applied to a zone IV to VII extensor tendon repair to a single digit or multiple digits. If all digits are involved, the ICAM regimen cannot be applied. It involves a combination of 2 custom-fabricated orthotic components that are much easier to create and comfortable to wear than other options. Howell and colleagues[46] referred to this regimen as a "relative motion protocol." They believed that the extensor tendons were reduced to a single motor unit system and therefore relaxed tension on the repair site. In a study supported by cadaveric data and 140 intraoperative cases, Howell and colleagues[46] found the ICAM resulted in 96% excellent and 93% good results. The ICAM has been found to work better with immediate referral within the first week after repair. The ICAM regimen has been modified over the years but consists of 3 distinct phases.

Phase 1 begins with referral to the hand therapy clinic within the first week for wound care, edema control, and custom orthosis fabrication. The orthosis is worn full time (**Table 4**). Active composite digital flexion and extension exercises are completed within the confines of the orthosis. The goal for this phase is full available digital active range of motion. Phase 2 begins after 21 days and continues through the fifth week. During this phase, the wrist component is discharged. The

patient continues the wearing the distal orthosis. The wrist component discharge can be delayed if the patient has activities that require heavy use of the hand. Active wrist motion is introduced with relaxed digits. The digits are gradually included with increased tension, with the goal of a composite wrist and digital active range of motion. Phase 3 begins after the fifth week and continues through the seventh week. The distal orthosis is used during the day. The orthosis is removed to exercise actively. Composite wrist and digital motion exercises are continued outside the orthosis. The distal orthosis may be discharged once full composite wrist and digital active range of motion are achieved (**Fig. 9**).

Many protocols are created or existing information is amended in the presence of consistent complications. Eissens and colleagues[47] experienced problems with extensor lags and the need for wrist level tenodesis surgery. They used the traditional zone V to VII static forearm-based orthosis with dynamic digital traction and wrist mobilization. The wrist is positioned in 25° of extension. The MPs are positioned at 0° with a flexion block at 30°. The PIP and DIP joints are free. The wrist motion is ingeniously achieved by removing the wrist strap and, during initial fabrication, creating a proximal strap that has a longer tag end. The tag end is repositioned to allow for the

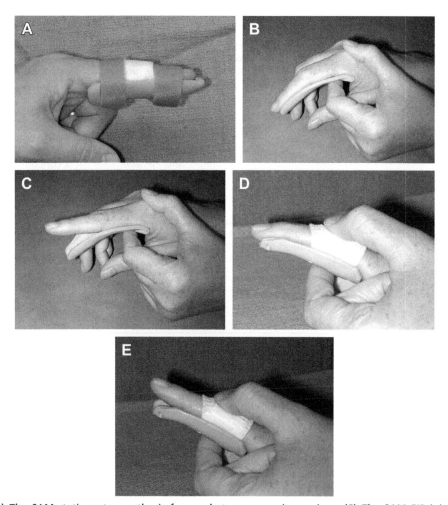

Fig. 8. (*A*) The SAM static custom orthosis for use between exercise sessions. (*B*) The SAM PIP joint exercise orthosis. Initially the wrist should be in 30° of extension and the MP in 0° to slight flexion. (*C*) The SAM PIP joint exercise should include full range of extension and flexion within the template limit. When the patient reaches full digital extension, they should gently and briefly hold the position. (*D*) The DIP template orthosis should allow for full flexion unless the lateral bands have been repaired. 30° to 35° is the appropriate block respecting the lateral band repair. (*E*) It is essential that the patient holds the PIP joint in 0° extension during the DIP joint exercises.

wrist to flex 20° in zones V and VI. For zone VII injuries, the wrist is allowed 15° of flexion. Wrist exercises are completed 10 times per waking hour and then the orthosis straps are returned to the original format. The author uses 2 pieces of sticky back hook, adheres them together, and places the hook on the proximal strap end opposite the tag end. This stops the tag end from flopping around as the patient engages in their ADLs. A second orthosis is fabricated to keep the digits in extension at night.

At postoperative day 3 to 5, the patient begins the protocol. For the first 3 weeks, the patient completes active digital flexion with passive flexion. The wrist exercises are completed in the orthosis with the digits in extension. The orthosis is modified at 3.5 weeks to increase available MP flexion to 50°. Modified place and hold exercises are completed with each digit separately, all digits together. The patient then completes active hook fists. All initial exercises are completed as well during this time frame. The orthosis is refabricated to allow for 70° of MP flexion. Active extension exercises are now completed with each digit separately, all digits simultaneously, hook fisting, and full composite fisting. Active wrist exercises through the full active plane are initiated with the digits in full passive extension. All previous exercises are completed as well. The sixth week signals the end of dynamic orthotic use. Night

Table 4
Dorsal blocking orthoses

Regimen	Wrist Position	MP Joint	Interphalangeal Joint	Special Considerations
SAM zones III and IV[43–45]	Exercise position 30° of wrist extension	Exercise position slight flexion or 0°	Static orthosis volar gutter with the PIP and DIP in extension 2 exercise orthoses: 1. PIP at 30° and DIP at 20°–25° 2. DIP at full flexion and PIP at 0°	The PIP template orthosis is progressed to 40° (2 wk), 50° (4 wk), and 60°–70° (end of week 4). 90° by 6 wk In the presence of a concomitant lateral band repair, the DIP orthosis is blocked at 30°–35° flexion
ICAM zones IV–VII[47]	30° extension	Repaired digit(s) blocked to 45° flexion	Free	Therapist fabricates 2 orthoses to work in tandem at initial visit Discontinue wrist component at 5 wk Discontinue digital component at 7 wk
Eissan et al protocol zones V–VII[48]	25° extension	Flexion block at 30° Dynamic traction brings digits back to 0° (no hyperextension) 3.5 wk: flexion block to 50°	Free (wrist exercises: zone VII blocked at 15° wrist flexion and 20° wrist flexion blocked at zones V and VI)	Distal wrist strap is removed completely and the proximal strap is reapplied to create a 20° flexion block to the wrist, during wrist exercises Night orthosis with digits in extension also fabricated
Double reverse Kleinert zones VI–VIII[49]	20°–30° wrist extension	0°–30° of flexion allowed	Free	No composite wrist and digital flexion Wrist is advanced 10° each week MP joints are advanced at 15° a week

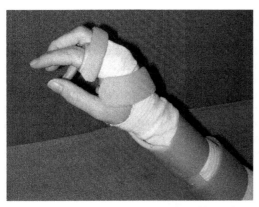

Fig. 9. The ICAM orthosis is a comfortable orthoses and is easy to make.

orthosis continues to be used. Composite wrist and digital active range of motion exercises and light PREs are added to the protocol. The patient may be ready for their full work capability around the tenth week (**Fig. 10**A–D).

Chinchalkar and Young[48] described a custom-fabricated dynamic orthosis they called the double reverse Kleinert extension splint. This orthosis includes a dynamic wrist component in conjunction with a digital dynamic component to apply controlled stress to repairs in zones VI to VIII. Its inception was a reaction to the complications encountered in zones VI to VIII. This protocol is included here to illustrate how far we have come in our journey to apply controlled stress to tendon repairs.

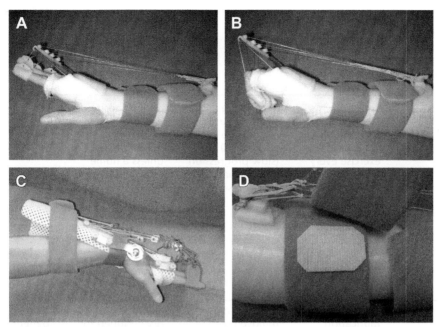

Fig. 10. (*A*) The dynamic orthosis allows for passive finger extension. However, hyperextension posturing should be avoided. (*B*) The active composite digital flexion within the limits of the flexion block is completed in the orthosis with passive extension. (*C*) The orthosis is adjusted to provide a restricted noncomposite wrist flexion exercise to 20°. (*D*) The authors use a doubled piece of hook to secure the extra long tag end.

There are no outcome studies available to advocate superiority of the use of this protocol. The protocol was vague as written. The patient has a custom double reverse Kleinert orthosis fabricated their during their first postoperative visit. This protocol needs to be implemented early after surgery. The wrist is positioned it seems in 20° to 30° of extension and 0°to 10° of flexion is allowed. The MP joints are positioned at 0° and are blocked with line stops to 30° of flexion. The patient is not to flex the wrist and digits together. The wrist is advanced at 10° each week. The MPs are advanced at 15° each week. This formula would allow for roughly 30° of wrist flexion and 90° of MP flexion at 6 weeks. Further research and information in the form of outcome studies are necessary (**Fig. 11**).

The common denominator between the flexor and extensor tendon regimens are controlled stress on the repair site. Surgeons, and more recently therapists, have been attempting to improve tendon excursion, decrease adhesions, and avoid complications since Sterling Bunnell watched his tendon repairs lose excursion progressively in the weeks after surgery.[51] The ever-evolving body of evidence continues to improve knowledge, techniques, and technology. This article has described a snapshot of early motion regimens for flexor and extensor tendons. The clinical decision-making process between the surgeon and therapist must assign or create the proper protocol to reduce the possibility of a poor result. The best surgical techniques can be beset with failure if the proper therapeutic management

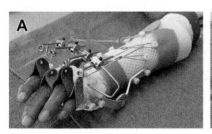
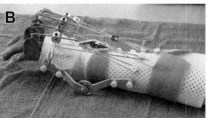

Fig. 11. (*A*) The double reverse Kleinert with digital and wrist dynamic components. (*B*) This orthosis is pictured without line stops or the wrist hinge stops.

Table 5
Extensor tendon early motion regimens

Extensor Tendon Early Motion Regimens	Initial to 2.5 wk	3.5–5wk	5–6 wk	6–8 wk
SAM zones III and IV	Orthoses fabrication Use template orthoses to exercise every waking hour for 20 repetitions each Hold wrist in 30° extension for exercise 2 wk: PIP template orthosis is refabricated to 40° PIP flexion	3 wk: change PIP angle to 50° 4 wk: change PIP angle to 70°–80° (slow progression if extensor lag is present)	5 wk: composite exercises and light PREs Discontinue at 6 wk unless a home exercise program has been reported	
ICAM zones IV–VII	Orthoses fabrication Full AROM within the confines of the orthosis Goal: full digital AROM	Proximal component removed for exercises and light ADL tasks Distal orthosis remains in full-time use At-risk tasks, the proximal portion is donned Noncomposite wrist AROM exercises with eventual addition of the digits by phase 3 Goal: complete composite digital and wrist AROM	Proximal portion is discontinued for all tasks Distal orthosis is removed for exercise but remains in use throughout the day	Discontinued by patient often around 7 wk Distal orthosis discontinued When full composite wrist and digital AROM are achieved
Eissan et al protocol zones V–VII	Dynamic orthosis fabricated 10 active repetitions of MP flexion blocked at 30° Active noncomposite wrist flexion exercises with digital joint full passive extension Zone V and VI 20° Zone VII 15°	Orthosis modified Continue previous exercises Place and hold exercises Hook fist	Orthosis modified Continue previous exercises Active extension and flexion to individual digits and as a group Hook fist Active composite fisting attempted Active wrist extension with digits in passive extension throughout repetitions	Orthosis discontinued Night orthosis worn Continue previous exercises Active wrist motion through full range Composite wrist and digital flexion/extension Light PREs 10+ wk: full use of the hand cleared

(continued on next page)

Table 5
(continued)

Extensor Tendon Early Motion Regimens	Initial to 2.5 wk	3.5–5wk	5–6 wk	6–8 wk
Double reverse Kleinert zones VI–VIII	Orthosis fabrication Active flexion of digits blocked at 30° flexion Active wrist flexion exercises blocked at 10°	Continue protocol advancement	Wrist block at 30° of wrist flexion Digital block at 90° of MP flexion	More information necessary regarding this protocol

Abbreviation: AROM, active range of motion.

is not initiated and managed properly. Independent study and a clinical dialogue with the patient care team is therefore encouraged to increase the functional outcomes for the patients and restore their activities (see **Table 4**; **Table 5**).

SUMMARY

An ideal protocol improves gliding of a repaired tendon, avoids repair rupture or gapping potential, and leads to a better functional return. After flexor tendon repair, early passive digital flexion regime is used popularly. Early active digital flexion is advocated increasingly in recent years following a strong tendon repair and possibly results in better recovery.[52–58] Following extensor tendon repair, some therapists and surgeons use early mobilization, but others use passive motion or immobilization. Whether the extensor tendon should be moved actively or passively, or immobilized, is controversial.[58,59] Application of the "right" force to move the digits is important to moving the repaired tendon while avoiding repair rupture. "Proper" positioning of the joints is important to reducing tension in the tendon. Limited active flexion and short dorsal blocking orthosis distal to the wrist are 2 recent advancements in flexor tendon rehabilitation. Most surgeons now prefer to initiate motion exercises 4–6 days after surgery. A variety of protocols are available currently. The decision of using a specific protocol is made for individual patients, and these protocols are often modified in their use to the patients, according to the extent of trauma to the tendon, strength of the tendon repair, and compliance of the patient.

REFERENCES

1. Duran R, Houser R. Controlled passive motion following flexor tendon repairing zones 2 and 3. In: Hunter JM, Schneider LH, editors. AAOS symposium on tendon surgery in the hand. St Louis (MO): CV Mosby; 1975. p. 105–14.
2. Kleinert HE, Kutz JE, Cohen MJ. Primary repair of zone 2 flexor tendon lacerations. In: Hunter JM, Schneider LH, editors. AAOS symposium on tendon surgery in the hand. St Louis (MO): CV Mosby; 1975. p. 105–14.
3. Strickland JW. Flexor tendon injuries II. Operative Treatment. J Am Acad Orthop Surg 1995;3:55–62.
4. Becker H, Graham MF, Cohen JK, et al. Intrinsic tendon cell proliferation in tissue culture. J Hand Surg Am 1981;6:616–93.
5. Gelberman RH, Steinberg D, Amiel D, et al. The early stages of flexor tendon healing: a morphologic study of the first fourteen days. J Hand Surg Am 1985;10:776–84.
6. Mass D, Tuel RJ. Intrinsic healing of the laceration site in human superficialis flexor tendons in vitro. J Hand Surg Am 1991;16:24–30.
7. Mass DP, Tuel RJ. Participation of human superficialis flexor tendon segments in repair in vitro. J Orthop Res 1990;8:21–34.
8. Strickland JW. Scientific basis for advances in flexor tendon surgery. J Hand Ther 2005;18:94–110.
9. Manske PR. Flexor tendon healing. J Hand Surg Br 1988;13:237–45.
10. Seyfer AE, Bolger WE. Effects of unrestricted motion on healing: a study of posttraumatic adhesions in primate tendons. Plast Reconstr Surg 1989;83:122–8.
11. Halikis MN, Manske PR, Kubota HM, et al. Effect of immobilization, immediate mobilization, and delayed mobilization on the resistance to digital flexion using a tendon injury model. J Hand Surg Am 1997;22:464–72.
12. Savage R. The influence of wrist position on the minimum force required for active movement of the interphalangeal joints. J Hand Surg Br 1988;13:262–8.

13. Urbaniak JR, Cahill JD Jr, Mortenson RA. Tendon suturing methods: analysis of tensile strengths. In: Hunter JM, Schneider LH, editors. AAOS symposium on tendon surgery in the hand. St Louis (MO): Mosby; 1975. p. 105–14.

14. Savage R. In vitro studies of a new flexor tendon repair. J Hand Surg Br 1985;10:135–41.

15. Choueka MD, Heminger H, Mass DP. Cyclical testing of zone II tendon repairs. J Hand Surg Am 2000;25:1127–34.

16. Miller L, Mass DP. A comparison of four repair techniques for camper's chiasma flexor digitorium superficialis lacerations: tested in an in vitro model. J Hand Surg Am 2000;25:1122–6.

17. Bassem E, Moran SL, Bravo C, et al. Factors that influence the outcome of zone 1 & 2 flexor tendon repairs in children. J Hand Surg Am 2006;31: 1661–6.

18. Tanaka T, Amadio PC, Zhao C, et al. Flexor digitorum profundus tendon tension during finger manipulation. J Hand Ther 2005;18:330–8.

19. Strickland JW, Glogovac SV. Digital function following flexor tendon repair in zone II: a comparison study of immobilization and controlled passive range of motion. J Hand Surg Am 1980;5:537–43.

20. Groth GN. Current practice patterns of flexor tendon rehabilitation. J Hand Ther 2005;18:169–74.

21. Cannon NM, editor. Diagnosis and treatment manual for physicians and therapists. 4th editon. Indianapolis (IN): The Hand Rehabilitation Center; 2001.

22. Pettengill KM, van Strien GV. Postoperative management of flexor tendon injuries. In: Skirven TM, Osterman AL, Fedorczyk JM, et al, editors. Rehabilitation of the hand and upper extremity, vol. 1, 6th edition. Philadelphia: Elsevier Mosby; 2011. p. 457–78.

23. Vucekovich K, Gallardo G, Fiala K. Rehabilitation after flexor tendon repair reconstruction and tenolysis. Hand Clin 2005;21:257–65.

24. Korstanje JW, Soeters JN, Schreuders TA, et al. Ultrasonographic assessment of flexor tendon mobilization: effect of different protocols on tendon excursion. J Bone Joint Surg Am 2012; 94:394–402.

25. Pettengill KM. The evolution of early mobilization of the repaired flexor tendon. J Hand Ther 2005;18: 157–68.

26. Cannon N. Post flexor tendon repair motion protocol. Indiana Hand Center Newsletter 1993;1:13–7.

27. Gratton P. Early active mobilization after flexor tendon repairs. J Hand Ther 1993;6:285–9.

28. Silfverskiöld KL, May EJ, Tornvall AH. Flexor digitorum profundus tendon excursions during controlled motion after flexor tendon repair in zone II: a prospective clinical study. J Hand Surg Am 1992;17:122–31.

29. Silfverskiold KL, May EJ, Tornvall AH. Tendon excursions after flexor tendon repair in zone II: results with a new controlled motion program. J Hand Surg Am 1993;18:403–10.

30. Small JO, Brennen MD, Colville J. Early active mobilization following flexor tendon repair in zone 2. J Hand Surg Br 1989;14:383–91.

31. Klien L. Early active motion flexor tendon protocol using one splint. J Hand Ther 2003;16:199–206.

32. Osada D, Fujita S, Tamai K, et al. Flexor tendon repair in zone II with 6-strand techniques and early active mobilization. J Hand Surg Am 2006; 31:987–92.

33. Wilhelmi BJ, Kang RH, Wages DJ, et al. Optimizing independent finger flexion with zone 5 flexor repairs using the Massachusetts General Hospital tenorrhaphy and early protected active motion. J Hand Surg Am 2005;30:230–6.

34. Tang JB. Indications, methods, postoperative motion and outcome evaluation of primary flexor tendon repairs in zone 2. J Hand Surg Eur 2007; 32:118–29.

35. Horii E, Lin GT, Cooney WP, et al. Comparative flexor tendon excursion after passive mobilization: an in vitro study. J Hand Surg Am 1992;17: 559–66.

36. Coats RW, Echevarria-Ore JC, Mass DP. Acute flexor tendon repairs in zone II. Hand Clin 2005; 21:173–9.

37. Greenwald D, Shumway S, Allen C, et al. Dynamic analysis of profundus tendon function. J Hand Surg Am 1994;19:626–35.

38. Evans RB. Rehabilitation techniques for applying immediate active tension to zone I and II flexor tendon repairs. Tech Hand Up Extrem Surg 1997; 1:286–96.

39. Clancy SP. Early active flexor tendon protocols. In: Diao E, Mass DP, editors. Tendon injuries in the hand and upper extremity: a master skills publication. Rosemont (IL): American Society of Surgery of the Hand; 2011. p. 273–85.

40. Trumble TE, Vedder NB, Seiler JG 3rd, et al. Zone-II flexor tendon repair: a randomized prospective trial of active place-and-hold therapy compared with passive motion therapy. J Bone Joint Surg Am 2010;92:1381–9.

41. Sandow MJ, McMahon M. Single-cross grasp six-strand repair for acute flexor tenorrhaphy: modified savage technique. In: Taras JS, Schnieder LH, editors. Atlas hand clinics. Philadelphia: Saunders; 1996. p. 41–64.

42. Sandow MJ, McMahon M. Active mobilization following single cross grasp four-strand flexor tenorrhaphy (Adelaide repair). J Hand Surg Eur 2011;36:467–75.

43. Evans RB. Clinical management of extensor tendon injuries: the therapist's perspective. In: Skirven TM,

Osterman AL, Fedorczyk JM, et al, editors. Rehabilitation of the hand and upper extremity, vol. 1, 6th edition. Philadelphia: Elsevier Mosby; 2011. p. 521–68.

44. Evans RB, Thompson DE. An analysis of factors that support early active short arc motion of the repaired central slip. J Hand Ther 1992;5:187–201.

45. Evans RB. Early active short arc motion for the repaired central slip. J Hand Surg Am 1994;19: 991–7.

46. Howell JW, Merritt WH, Robinson SJ. Immediate controlled active motion following zone 4–7 extensor tendon repair. J Hand Ther 2005;18:182–90.

47. Eissens MH, Shut SM, van der Sluis CK. Early active wrist mobilization in extensor tendon injuries in zones 5, 6, or 7. J Hand Ther 2007;20: 89–91.

48. Chinchalkar S, Young SA. A double reverse Kleinert extension splint for extensor tendon repairs in zones VI to VIII. J Hand Ther 2004;17:424–6.

49. Evans RB, Thompson DE. The application of force to the healing tendon. J Hand Ther 1993;6: 266–84.

50. Aurand ED, Thomas E. Rehabilitation of extensor tendon injuries. In: Diao E, Mass DP, editors. Tendon injuries in the hand and upper extremity: a master skills publication. Rosemont (IL): American Society of Surgery of the Hand; 2011. p. 273–85.

51. Bunnell S. Repair of tendons in the fingers and description of two new instruments. Surg Gynecol Obstet 1918;26:103–10.

52. Tang JB. Clinical outcomes associated with flexor tendon repair. Hand Clin 2005;21:199–210.

53. Lee SK. Modern tendon repair techniques. Hand Clin 2012;28:565–70.

54. Wu YF, Cao Y, Zhou YL, et al. Biomechanical comparisons of four-strand tendon repairs with double-stranded sutures: effects of different locks and suture geometry. J Hand Surg Eur 2011;36:34–9.

55. Orkar KS, Watts C, Iwuagwu FC. A comparative analysis of the outcome of flexor tendon repair in the index and little fingers: Does the little finger fare worse? J Hand Surg Eur 2012;37:20–6.

56. Yamazaki H, Kato H, Uchiyama S, et al. Long term results of early active extension and passive flexion mobilization following one-stage tendon grafting for neglected injuries of the flexor digitorum profundus in children. J Hand Surg Eur 2011;36:303–7.

57. Ruchelsman DE, Christoforou D, Wasserman B, et al. Avulsion injuries of the flexor digitorum profundus tendon. J Am Acad Orthop Surg 2011;19: 152–62.

58. Tang JB. Tendon injuries across the world: treatment. Injury 2006;37:1036–42.

59. Howell JW, Peck F. Rehabilitation of flexor and extensor tendon injuries in the hand: Current updates. Injury 2013;44:397–402.

Editors' Note:
Intrinsic Tendon Healing and Staged Tendon Reconstruction: Reflection of Legends

Hand surgeons are familiar with intrinsic tendon healing capacity and staged tendon reconstruction. Dr. James M. Hunter pioneered the procedures of staged tendon reconstruction, and the seminal investigations of synovial nutrition of the tendon made by Dr. Paul R. Manske provided fundamental experimental evidence that led to the recognition of the intrinsic healing capacity of tendon.

Dr. Hunter's staged tendon reconstruction remains an important procedure in today's practice, and Dr. Manske's investigations in tendon healing remains a cornerstone of current primary digital flexor tendon repair.

At the time of completion of editing this issue of *Hand Clinics*, devoted to "Tendon Repair and Reconstruction," we pay particular tribute to the 2 pioneering surgeons—Drs. James M. Hunter (1924–2013) and Paul R. Manske (1938–2011)—dedicated surgeons, legendary editors, pioneers, great teachers, and friends to many of us.

"Reflection of Legends" was a theme of a major session at the Congress of the International Federation of Societies for Surgery of the Hand last month. The ingenious investigations of tendon repair and reconstruction made by both surgeons are a reflection of their legendary careers.

Staged tendon reconstruction and investigations in the tendon healing mechanism are perfectly exemplary of the impact and needs of both technical innovation and basic science advancement in the field of hand surgery.

Jin Bo Tang, MD

Steve K. Lee, MD

Hand Clin 29 (2013) 311
http://dx.doi.org/10.1016/j.hcl.2013.04.001
0749-0712/13/$ – see front matter © 2013 Published by Elsevier Inc.

Index

Note: Page numbers of article titles are in **boldface** type.

Moving?

Make sure your subscription moves with you!

To notify us of your new address, find your **Clinics Account Number** (located on your mailing label above your name), and contact customer service at:

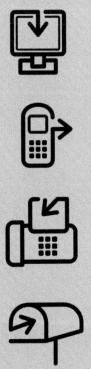

Email: journalscustomerservice-usa@elsevier.com

800-654-2452 (subscribers in the U.S. & Canada)
314-447-8871 (subscribers outside of the U.S. & Canada)

Fax number: 314-447-8029

Elsevier Health Sciences Division
Subscription Customer Service
3251 Riverport Lane
Maryland Heights, MO 63043

*To ensure uninterrupted delivery of your subscription, please notify us at least 4 weeks in advance of move.

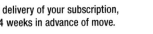

Printed and bound by CPI Group (UK) Ltd, Croydon, CR0 4YY

03/10/2024

01040344-0010